Eating Well,
Staying Well
During and After Cancer

Eating Well, Staying Well
During and After Cancer

Edited by

Abby Bloch, PhD, RD
Barrie R. Cassileth, PhD
Michelle D. Holmes, MD, DrPH
Cynthia A. Thomson, PhD, RD

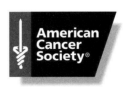

Published by
American Cancer Society
Health Promotions
1599 Clifton Road NE
Atlanta, Georgia 30329, USA

Printed in the United States of America
Recipe analyses provided by the University of Arizona Cancer Center, Nutrition and Behavior Measurement Unit.

5 4 3 2 1   03 04 05 06 07

Library of Congress Cataloging-in-Publication Data

Eating well, staying well during and after cancer / Abby Bloch ...
[et al.].
        p. cm.
Includes bibliographical references and index.
    ISBN 0-944235-51-4 (pbk. : alk. paper)
    1. Cancer--Nutritional aspects. 2. Cancer--Diet therapy. I.
Bloch, Abby S.

    RC268.45.E285 2003
    616.99'40654--dc22
                                                    2003016748

A Note to the Reader

The information contained in this book is not intended as medical advice and should not be relied upon as a substitute for talking with your doctor. This information may not address all possible actions, precautions, side effects, or interactions. All matters regarding your health require the supervision of a medical doctor who is familiar with your medical needs. For more information, contact your American Cancer Society at 800-ACS-2345 or *www.cancer.org*.

About the Editors

Abby Bloch, PhD, RD

Bloch is the former chair of the American Cancer Society Nutrition and Physical Activity Advisory Committee. An associate professor at the New York University Graduate School and at the University of Medicine and Dentistry of New Jersey and a nutrition consultant in private practice in New York, she has published four books and numerous chapters in textbooks, journals, and other publications relating to nutrition and prevention, wellness, cancer management, and clinical aspects of nutrition and diet. She serves on the Complementary and Alternative Methods Advisory Workgroup for the American Cancer Society and is an associate professor at New York University graduate school and University of Medicine and Dentistry of New Jersey.

Barrie R. Cassileth, PhD

The chief of integrative medicine service at Memorial Sloan-Kettering Cancer Center's Integrative Medicine Center, Cassileth is the author of a book on complementary and alternative therapies (CAM) and has published numerous chapters in oncology textbooks and articles in top medical journals. She has written a monthly column in the Los Angeles Times on CAM topics; served on the National Institutes of Health (NIH) Advisory Panel on Unconventional Medical Practices for five years; and was a founding member of the Advisory Council to the National Institutes of Health Office of Alternative Medicine in 1994. She has been a member of the national Board of Directors of the American Cancer Society since 1998, and she serves on several ACS committees relating to CAM therapies and health policy.

Michelle D. Holmes, MD, DrPH

Holmes is assistant professor of Medicine at Harvard Medical School and is an epidemiologist at Channing Laboratory at Brigham and Women's Hospital. She practiced primary care internal medicine for 18 years, caring for a number of people with cancer and their families. She is now an epidemiological researcher examining diet and cancer. Her research interests include the dietary determinants of cancer and lifestyle factors (including diet) that may possibly affect the longevity and quality of life of people with cancer.

Cynthia A. Thomson, PhD, RD

Thomson is assistant professor of nutritional sciences at the University of Arizona and is a researcher at the Arizona Cancer Center. She is currently the Arizona site lead investigator on three national studies looking at the role of diet in breast cancer prevention. She provides support for cancer patients through community outreach programs, through the Arizona Cancer Center Nutrition Ways web site, and as a clinician and educator. She is a recent rectal cancer survivor.

EDITORIAL REVIEW
Terri Ades, RN, MS, AOCN
Patti Breitman
Tim Byers, MD, MPH
Joy Fincannon Carter, RN, MS
Colleen Doyle, MS, RD
Ted Gansler, MD, MBA
Greta Greer, LCSW, CCM
Marilyn Majchrzak, MS, RD
Marji McCullough, ScD, RD
Diane B. Wilson, EdD, MS, RD

MANAGING EDITOR
Gianna Marsella, MA

EDITOR
Amy Brittain

BOOK PUBLISHING MANAGER
Candace Magee

PUBLISHING DIRECTOR
Diane Scott-Lichter, MA

EDITORIAL AND
NEW MEDIA DIRECTOR
David Ragals

DIRECT CHANNELS
MANAGING DIRECTOR
Chuck Westbrook

Acknowledgments

We would like to gratefully acknowledge the generous contributions of the dozens of American Cancer Society volunteers and other individuals who provided valuable tips, photographs, and nutritious recipe suggestions. Without their help and the benefit of their experience, this book would not have been possible.

Contents

Chapter 4 • Food Quality and Safety   45

Chapter 5 • Dietary Supplements: Vitamins, Minerals, and Herbs   55

Section Two

How Can My Diet Help Me Stay Strong during Treatment?

Section Three
How Should I Eat after Treatment Is Over?

Section Four

Easy Meals to Rely on during and after Treatment

How Are Nutrition and Cancer Related?

A CANCER DIAGNOSIS CAN IMPACT EVERYTHING—including your priorities, your family life, and your outlook. While you're learning about many important aspects of cancer and cancer treatment, from treatment choices to work and family needs, what to eat may be the furthest thing from your mind. But eating well is more important than ever when you're undergoing cancer treatment.

Nutrition and Cancer

Eating a healthful diet during and after your treatment can help you:

- feel better
- keep up your strength and energy
- keep up your weight and your body's store of nutrients
- tolerate treatment-related side effects
- maximize the benefits of treatment
- decrease your risk of infection
- heal and recover quickly

Studies show that patients who eat well during cancer treatment are better able to tolerate chemotherapy, radiation therapy, surgery, or biological therapy side effects. People who eat well during cancer treatment may even be able to tolerate higher doses of treatments.

Proper nutrition continues to be essential during recovery from treatment and in life after cancer, as well as for those living with advanced cancer.

Cancer Nutrition Information

Advice about what to eat when you have cancer is everywhere—which foods help or hinder cancer treatment, diets that are presented as cancer cures, and how to eat if you're experiencing side effects from treatment. You may already have heard and read all kinds of information from fellow cancer patients, friends, on the Internet, and in books. Some advice—such as that you receive from your health care team—is likely to be accurate and helpful; other suggestions may not help and may even be dangerous. How do you know where to start?

The search for information about cancer nutrition can be a challenge. At times, even respected sources offer conflicting information. There may not be solid evidence about a particular issue, which confuses matters. In *Eating Well, Staying Well During and After Cancer*, the experts at the American Cancer Society will introduce you to some of the important issues and facts about diet and cancer. Your doctor, dietitian, and nurse can evaluate your situation and help you decide which options may work best for you.

RELY ON YOUR HEALTH CARE TEAM

Each person's body, cancer, and reactions to treatment will be different. Members of your health care team—your doctor, dietitian, and nurse—are an invaluable resource and can help you navigate through information about nutrition. They can help you put together an eating plan that takes into account your cancer, your treatment, any side effects you experience, and your levels of immunity and energy. Listening to your body and paying attention to what it's telling you will also help shape your nutrition plan to maximize your quality of life and your health.

Your health care team should be able to provide referrals to other experts or researchers if you want additional opinions or nutritional advice.

You may be considering integrating supplements or complementary therapies into your treatment. Seek the advice of your health care team and let them know if you plan to use any supplements or complementary therapies so they can determine any interactions that could interfere with treatment. ***Using alternative treatments instead of standard cancer treatments is not recommended; discuss any plan to use alternative therapies in the place of standard treatments with your doctor.***

How This Book Is Organized

This book is designed for people with cancer and their families and other care-givers. It's organized so you can browse through it and read the sections that fit your current situation. Later you can read other sections as you need them. If you are one of the cancer patients who does experience eating-related treatment side effects during or after treatment, you may first want to read the sections explaining how to cope with them. If you have no side effects or only mild side effects, you may find that the chapters about nutrition before treatment; foods, vitamins and minerals, herbs, and diets promoted as cures for cancer; and nutrition after treatment and for long-term wellness will be most useful.

Section 1: How Can My Diet Affect My Cancer Treatment?

What you need to know before cancer treatment begins about what to eat and what to avoid to stay strong, including:

- **Chapter 1, What Healthful Eating Means:** Nutrients needed for healthful eating before treatment, why nutritional needs may be different for people with cancer, and how to research claims, understand study types, and interpret information about nutrition and cancer.

- **Chapter 2, Vegetables, Fruits, and Whole Grains:** Information about produce as well as specific vegetables and fruits and how they affect the body, nutrients retained in raw and cooked produce, and an explanation of the glycemic index.

- **Chapter 3, Foods of Special Interest:** Foods of special interest to people with cancer because of attention—whether deserved or undeserved— paid to them as being helpful for those in cancer treatment or those hoping to reduce cancer risk.

- **Chapter 4, Food Quality and Safety:** Information about genetically modified foods, irradiated foods, organic foods, pesticides, food additives, and how they affect those with cancer and those who have had cancer.

- **Chapter 5, Dietary Supplements: Vitamins, Minerals, and Herbs:** Dietary supplements, risks of drug interactions, how to research them and talk about your doctor with them, how they're regulated and manufactured, and how to understand claims and labels; the powerful effects of vitamins and minerals on your health, especially during treatment, and food sources for each vitamin and mineral.

- **Chapter 6, Diets Promoted as Cures for Cancer:** Diets presented as being cures or helpful for those with cancer; which might help your health, and which are dangerous and should be avoided.

Section 2: How Can My Diet Help Me Stay Strong during Treatment?

Practical ways to prepare physically and mentally for treatment and nutrition during treatment, and detailed information on common eating-related side effects that people experience with their treatment and how to cope with them.

- **Chapter 7, Eating or Digestion Challenges during Treatment:** How to get ready for treatment and nutrition suggestions for people undergoing surgery, radiation, chemotherapy, immunotherapy, and hormonal therapy.
- **Chapter 8, "I want to maintain my body weight."** Why you might experience weight loss or weight gain, and how to cope and maintain your weight.
- **Chapter 9, "I want to have more energy."** Why you might feel fatigued, how to cope with fatigue, and ways to boost your energy.
- **Chapter 10, "I want to improve my immunity."** How an altered immune system may affect your health during treatment and how to cope with it, including tips about food safety.
- **Chapter 11, "I want to stay hydrated."** Why you might become dehydrated during therapy and how to remain hydrated, including daily fluid needs and suggestions.
- **Chapter 12, "I want to cope with eating or digestion issues."** What to expect from and how to cope with other potential treatment side effects, such as nausea and vomiting, diarrhea, constipation, lactose intolerance, changes in taste or smell, loss of appetite, sore throat, dry mouth or thick saliva, mouth sores, and difficulty swallowing.

Section 3: How Should I Eat after Treatment Is Over?

What you can do to establish a pattern of healthful eating after treatment and for the rest of your life.

- **Chapter 13, Eating Well Every Day:** How to get back into healthful eating and physical activity: their roles in a healthful lifestyle and their effects on cancer recurrence.

Section 4: Easy Meals to Rely on during and after Treatment

- **Recipe Resource Section: Simple, Healthful Recipes for the Whole Family:** Menus and recipes that are easy and healthful enough to rely on before, during, and after treatment, including some recipes straight from cancer survivors' kitchens. Recipe analyses were provided by the University of Arizona Cancer Center, Nutrition and Behavior Measurement Unit.

Other Sections

- **Resources:** Organizations and resources that provide information and services for people with cancer.
- **Glossary:** Key terms and definitions related to nutrition and living well both during and after cancer.
- **References:** A list of sources for the information in this book.

Two important sections that appear throughout the book are:

- **On the Horizon:** In these short sections, we delve into exciting new studies, discoveries, or research related to foods, herbs, and other nutrition-related factors that may have important implications related to cancer and its treatment. *On the Horizon* sections present preliminary research of interest and do not constitute recommendations.
- **Tips from people with cancer:** Men and women from across the country generously share their wisdom about eating, cooking, planning, and coping with challenges during cancer and its treatment. They offer tips big and small, general wellness plans, specific items to keep on hand, and their thoughts on keeping things in perspective. Many of them share the ways in which they made meals more pleasurable and what foods they enjoyed eating along the way. This advice will show you what worked and what didn't for others, so that you'll be able to test out methods and try out others' solutions.

The experts at the American Cancer Society outline issues you may want to consider while you're eating for health. *Eating Well, Staying Well During and After Cancer* will help you sift through advice for sound dietary information as you go through cancer treatment and beyond. We hope it will help you become better informed about the many options you have for eating and staying well and the issues being discussed and researched now. We also hope that the information here will lead you to ask your health care team questions about how these issues might apply to you and your situation.

About the American Cancer Society

The American Cancer Society is a nationwide community-based voluntary health organization. Represented in more than 3,400 communities throughout the United States and Puerto Rico, the American Cancer Society is dedicated to eliminating cancer as a major health problem. This book is just one example of the many ways the society seeks to fulfill its mission: to save lives and diminish suffering from cancer through research, education, advocacy, and service.

The American Cancer Society is the largest private source of cancer research dollars in the U.S. Founded in 1913 by ten physicians and five concerned members of the community, the organization is now represented by two million Americans. Most offer their time free of charge to the society to work to conquer cancer.

How Can My Diet Affect My Body and Its Response to Cancer Treatment?

Chapter 1

What Healthful Eating Means

WE ALL KNOW THAT EATING WELL is an important part of healthful lifestyle. But what do we mean by "eating well" or "healthful eating"? Eating well is simply eating a balance of foods to help maintain your health. Along with being physically active, keeping a healthful weight, and limiting the alcohol you drink, eating well is a powerful way to help your body stay strong.

What Healthful Eating Means to Someone with Cancer

Eating healthfully is essential for people with cancer. Getting the nutrients you need will help you fight cancer. Several nutrients may actually slow the growth of some types of cancer. More and more people are living long lives after cancer treatment, and balancing your diet and staying physically active make up a solid foundation for healthful living throughout your life.

We'll get into the details of what eating healthfully may mean specifically for you at different stages of cancer and its treatment in this chapter and throughout this book. In chapters 7 through 12, we'll outline eating to help cope with specific side effects, and in chapter 13, we'll talk about specific issues to keep in mind following treatment; for now, let's look at the diet that may help you before treatment.

What to Eat before Treatment

Before treatment, your goal is to stay strong so treatment can have the most positive effects possible. Talk to members of your health care team to find out if they have specific suggestions for your diet as you prepare for treatment. In general, following a sound plan for overall nutritional health is the best plan for you and your family whether cancer is present on not.

The principles outlined in the American Cancer Society (ACS) Guidelines on Nutrition and Physical Activity for Cancer Prevention (comparable to the recommendations of several other organizations, agencies, and expert panels for dietary foundations aimed at preventing cancer and other chronic diseases) are also cited by the American Cancer Society Expert Committee report, "Nutrition and Physical Activity During and After Cancer Treatment: A Guide for Informed Choices" as the basis for a healthful diet during all phases of the cancer experience:

- Eat five or more servings of a variety of vegetables and fruits each day.
- Choose whole grains in preference to processed (refined) grains and sugars.
- Limit consumption of red meats, especially those high in fat and processed.
- Choose foods that help you maintain a healthful weight.

For more information about vegetables, fruits, and whole grains, see chapter 2.

It's difficult to generalize about maintaining weight during treatment since some people may have specific needs even before treatment starts. If a person is underweight before treatment and a health care team recommends an intensive treatment that is likely to cause significant weight loss, that person may be advised to gain weight before treatment and concentrate on eating high-calorie foods. Talk to your health care team about the right plan for your situation.

Healthful Eating Tips

My best friend was diagnosed with breast cancer five years ago, at the age of 39. This event changed everything in her life—she had little control over her situation. Healthful eating is a positive life change and is something she could control. Inspired by my friend, I am happy to say that I have made healthy changes, I've lost 30 pounds, and I've maintained my ideal weight.

—Kristi

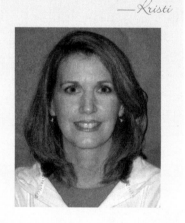

What counts as a serving?

Here's how the United States Department of Agriculture (USDA) defines a serving of fruit and vegetables (which is also what the National Cancer Institute recommends):

- 1 medium piece of fruit or ½ cup fruit
- ¾ cup (180 milliliters) of 100 percent juice
- ¼ cup dried fruit
- ½ cup raw non-leafy or cooked vegetables
- 1 cup raw leafy vegetables (such as lettuce)
- ½ cup cooked beans or peas (such as lentils, pinto beans, and kidney beans)

VEGETABLES AND FRUITS

It's reasonable for most people with cancer to follow dietary recommendations from the ACS and many other organizations for eating five or more daily servings of vegetables and fruits. Many items, such as baby carrots, grapes, cherry tomatoes, and bananas, can be eaten on the spot, with minimal preparation. (Fresh produce should be washed with water before eating to remove any surface dirt and bacteria, especially if you'll eat the skin.)

WHOLE GRAINS

Grains provide complex carbohydrates (starches), which help provide energy, fiber (the part of plant foods that the body cannot digest), and vitamins and minerals such as folate. Whole grains like barley, brown rice, whole wheat, or bulgur contain the whole grain or seed. Different whole-grain foods differ in nutrient content, but they provide more vitamins, minerals, fiber, and other protective substances than refined grains. Refined grains are stripped of the bran and germ during processing and are therefore low in fiber and in the protective substances that accompany fiber. A regular intake of fiber-rich foods such as whole grains (as well as many vegetables) helps maintain proper bowel function.

LIMIT RED MEAT

Red meat contains iron for the blood and proteins and fatty acids for growth, but it also often comes with a high amount of saturated fat and cholesterol.

A moderate amount of meats—especially lean cuts and smaller portions—along with fish, chicken, fruits, vegetables, whole grains, and healthy sources of fat, can make up a balanced diet. Baking, broiling, or poaching meat is more healthful than frying or charbroiling. Other ways to cut down on your intake of fats from meat include making meat a side dish rather than the main course and trimming the fats from meat prior to cooking.

BALANCE YOUR DIET

Eating a diverse diet that includes a variety of nutrients is the easiest way to make sure you're getting everything you need. It's important that everyone regularly eats a variety of nutrients, but it's especially crucial for people with cancer. Here's a quick rundown of the why, where, and when of the nutrients you'll need most. You'll find tips for incorporating these nutrients into your diet in chapter 7.

Keep in mind that there's a crucial difference between getting nutrients through food and taking supplements. While eating a balanced diet benefits your body, certain supplements—for example, the antioxidants vitamins C and E and folic acid—that provide concentrated nutrients *may interfere with the effectiveness of certain chemotherapy agents or with radiation therapy.* (For more information about supplements, see chapter 5.)

Proteins. Proteins provide the body with amino acids, which allow for growth, repair body tissue, maintain a healthy immune system, and play important roles in other functions of the body. They help build cells and create hormones and enzymes. Without enough protein, the body takes longer to recover from illness and lowers its resistance to infection.

People with cancer often need more protein than usual. Taking in additional protein after surgery, chemotherapy, and radiation therapy will help heal tissues and prevent infection. Getting enough protein is crucial not only during cancer treatment and recovery, but also after treatment. Ten percent or more calories from protein is typically adequate for adults (most elderly people need to take in additional calories from protein, and people with kidney problems may want to take in fewer calories from protein).

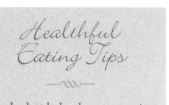

Healthful Eating Tips

I feel what helped me to survive treatment and breast cancer itself is eating well. Since childhood I've relied on fruits, vegetables, and grains and eat little or no fast food. It's a way of life in our family.

—*Janet*

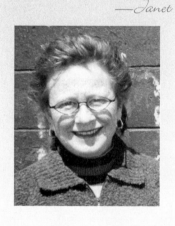

6

Good sources of protein include animal foods like lean meat, fish, poultry, and dairy products, as well as plant foods like nuts, dried beans, peas and lentils, and soy foods.

Carbohydrates. Carbohydrates supply the body with the bulk—50 to 60 percent—of the calories it needs to function. The amount of calories each person needs depends on age, size, and level of physical activity.

Carbohydrates will give you energy during cancer treatment. Breads, pasta, grains and cereal products, dried beans, peas, lentils, fruits, and vegetables are all sources of carbohydrates, which provide the body with quick energy, as well as other nutrients.

Sugars like honey, molasses, syrups, and white or brown sugar are sources of concentrated carbohydrates, which add calories to your diet but don't offer other nutrients. Foods high in refined (processed) sugars or carbohydrates may also intensify the body's resistance to insulin, a hormone naturally produced by the pancreas that allows the body to use sugar from food as an energy source. We don't know if this is important in cancer survival, but it likely factors into increasing obesity and raising the risk of diabetes and cardiovascular disease.

Choosing whole grains (such as whole-grain rice, bread, pasta, and cereals) over refined grains (like white bread and potatoes) and sugars (including pastries, sweetened cereals, soft drinks, and sugars) will give your body the carbohydrate energy it needs. (See the *Carbohydrates and the Glycemic Index* section of chapter 2 for more information.)

Fats. Fats provide the body with calories for physical activity as well as fatty acids that help the body grow, produce hormones, transport some vitamins, and build new cells. Fat also protects the organs of the body against trauma. The body stores excess calories as fat, which is saved up as reserve energy. This is important during cancer treatment.

There are three main types of fatty acids: saturated, monounsaturated, and polyunsaturated. Saturated fatty acids are mostly found in meats and whole-milk products. (Trans fatty acids, also called trans-saturated fats and trans fats, are not found in nature but are added to margarines,

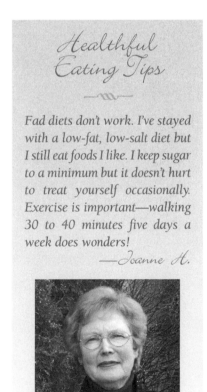

Healthful Eating Tips

Fad diets don't work. I've stayed with a low-fat, low-salt diet but I still eat foods I like. I keep sugar to a minimum but it doesn't hurt to treat yourself occasionally. Exercise is important—walking 30 to 40 minutes five days a week does wonders!
—*Joanne H.*

vegetable shortenings, and packaged breads, cakes, cookies, and crackers to give these products longer shelf lives. They are similar to saturated fat in that they raise blood cholestrol.)

Monounsaturated fatty acids and polyunsaturated fatty acids (either omega-3 or omega-6) are mostly found in plant foods like vegetables, nuts, and grains and their oils (such as canola, soybean, safflower, and corn oil), as well as in some seafood. Some studies show that eating foods that contain polyunsaturated and monounsaturated fats can reduce levels of LDL-cholesterol ("bad cholesterol") in the blood.

Saturated fats get a lot of attention as having a greater potential effect on increasing cancer risk than other types, while fats that contain omega-3 fatty acids (see chapter 3) are often called "good fats." The role of fat in cancer risk is controversial and continues to be studied.

Much of the interest in the possible effects of dietary fat on cancer risk has focused on breast cancer. In most studies, total fat intake has not been linked to a lower risk for breast cancer recurrence (cancer that comes back after treatment, whether in the same place as the original cancer, in the lymph nodes, or after spreading to another area of the body) or reduced survival. Two large clinical trials are examining the potential effect of dietary fat on breast cancer recurrence and survival (see the *Studying Nutrition and Recurrence* section on page 190 of chapter 13 for more information).

Fat provides more concentrated calories than carbohydrates or proteins, so eating more fat is an easy way to take in more calories when a person experiences digestion challenges during or after treatment and eats less. But greasy or oily foods may be hard to digest for people who are undergoing cancer treatment.

Vitamins. Vitamins help the body use energy (calories) from carbohydrates, fats, and proteins. Bone strength, vision, and skin, nails, and hair rely on the vitamins you eat.

A person who eats a balanced diet with enough calories and protein usually gets plenty of vitamins. However, eating a balanced diet can be challenging when you are receiving cancer treatment, particularly if treatment side effects continue for extended periods. During and after cancer treatment, taking a standard multiple vitamin and mineral supplement that contains approximately 100 percent of the recommended amounts is probably a healthful choice, since it may be difficult for you to eat enough micronutrients (dietary elements essential in small quantities for growth and health). Talk to your dietitian or doctor

Good Health Includes Weight Control

Preliminary findings of a recently published study showed that adolescents who regularly eat eggs, vegetable oils, and dietary fiber may grow up with a lower incidence of breast cancer than others. This study of 121,000 women is reinforcing what researchers have long suspected: that a teen's diet may affect her adult risk of breast cancer.

Eating about three eggs a week when a woman was 12 to 18 seemed to decrease her risk of breast cancer by almost 20 percent. (There is no evidence to show that doubling the number of eggs consumed will double a young woman's protection from breast cancer.) Eating vegetable oils and dietary fiber also lowered the breast cancer risk. (Eating approximately a teaspoon of butter a day increased the risk by over five percent.) Eggs are high in essential amino acids (organic compounds found in plants and animals that are the main components of protein), vitamins, and minerals, which may be responsible for the protective effect. High-fiber foods may decrease estrogen levels—and estrogen, a female hormone, helps the breast and some breast cancers grow.

The study relied on women's memories of their diets in adolescence, which is often difficult. These are preliminary findings, and young women shouldn't change their diets to concentrate on eggs, oil, and fiber—a balanced diet is still the healthiest way to give your body the nutrients it needs. Researchers will continue to study these foods to determine what, if any, the link is between these foods and breast cancer.

about a daily multivitamin/mineral supplement and whether it is appropriate for your situation. (See chapter 5 for more information about vitamins.)

Minerals. Minerals spur on and regulate the body's processes. Iron, for example, carries oxygen to your cells. Calcium helps your bones and teeth stay strong, and potassium helps nerves and muscles function.

Eating a variety of foods generally supplies your body with enough minerals. But cancer treatments such as surgery and chemotherapy may deplete the body's stores of vitamins and minerals. If you aren't taking in enough food to meet recommended daily allowances of minerals or are undergoing surgery or chemotherapy, talk to your health care team about strategies such as taking a multivitamin/mineral supplement. (See chapter 5 for more information about minerals.)

Water. Water and fluids are vital to health. They make up from half to two thirds of your total body weight. Water regulates the body's temperature, transports nutrients where they are needed, and removes waste.

If you do not take in enough fluids or if you are vomiting or have diarrhea during cancer treatment, you may become dehydrated. Unless you are directed to do otherwise, try to drink six to eight glasses of water a day. If you need to add calories to your diet, you can drink high-calorie liquids instead of water. Ask your doctor or nurse how much fluid you need each day to prevent dehydration. (See chapter 11 for more information about staying hydrated.)

RDAS, DRIS: KNOW THE LINGO

The Recommended Dietary Allowances (RDAs) have been published for over 60 years by the Food and Nutrition Board of the National Academy of Sciences (NAS). Our knowledge about nutrients and how nutrient levels affect individuals and groups has grown significantly since the RDAs were established. The RDAs are gradually being replaced with Dietary Reference Intakes (DRIs), which encompass four nutrient values:

- Recommended Dietary Allowance (RDA). The average daily dietary intake of a nutrient that meets the nutrition needs of nearly all (97 to 98 percent of) healthy individuals in a population.
- Adequate Intake (AI). When an RDA cannot be estimated for a nutrient, an AI is determined. AIs are developed based on observations about a group of healthy people's average intake of a nutrient. Individuals should rely on the AI as guide when no RDA is available.
- Tolerable Upper Intake Level (UL). The highest daily level of a nutrient that is likely to be safe for almost all individuals—that is, likely not to pose a risk of adverse health effects. This is not an ideal or a recommended intake level.
- Estimated Average Requirement (EAR). The amount of a nutrient that meets the estimated nutrient needs of half of all healthy individuals in a population. (EARs are used as a guide when RDAs are developed.)

The DRIs are nutrient level guides for both individuals (RDAs, AIs, and ULs) and groups (EARs). To make things more confusing, the Daily Values (DVs) of nutrients shown on current nutrition labels are based on U.S. RDAs—which are based on but are not exactly the same as the Food and Nutrition Board's RDAs. The Food and Drug Administration (FDA) developed the U.S. RDA system in the 1970s to take the place of the minimum daily nutrition requirements that were used until that time for labeling purposes.

RDAs (or AIs) will help you evaluate your appropriate average daily nutrient intake; use ULs as a guide to maximum safe intake levels for nutrients. Keep in mind that DRIs are nutrient estimates for healthy individuals. RDAs and AIs are average nutrient intake guidelines and may not be accurate recommendations for people with increased nutritional needs. Talk to your health care team about the level of nutrients you need at different stages of your cancer and treatment. (For more information about DRIs, visit the Institute of Medicine of the National Academy of Sciences Web site at *http://www.iom.edu*.)

Your Nutrition Plan and Goals

Good nutrition is especially important for people with cancer, but nutritional needs vary from person to person. People with cancer—especially those in treatment—often have increased and specific nutritional needs. Before you begin cancer treatment, you'll want to discuss with your health care team how you may be able to best ready yourself for treatment nutritionally. Your dietitian, doctor, and nurse can help tailor your eating plan to your health, your cancer type, and the treatment you'll receive and its expected effects on you. They can help identify your nutrition goals and can plan detailed strategies to help you meet them. You can also look to them for guidance in maintaining nutritional goals as you recover from treatment and in your life after cancer. (See page 17 of the *Talk to the Experts* section of this chapter for information about finding a dietitian.)

When you're healthy, eating enough food to get the nutrients you need is usually not a problem. Most nutrition guidelines stress eating lots of vegetables, fruits, and whole-grain products; consuming enough protein to meet your needs; consuming moderate amounts of low-fat meat and dairy foods; and cutting back on saturated fat, sugar, refined carbohydrates, alcohol, and salt.

During and after cancer treatment, however, getting enough nutrients may become a challenge, especially if you experience side effects or simply don't feel well. Your metabolism (the breaking down of molecules to make energy for the body), appetite, and your body's ability to tolerate certain foods and use nutrients may be affected by cancer and its treatments. As a result, you may have to change your diet to help you build up strength and withstand the effects of your cancer and its treatment.

Update: Diet and Cancer

People who have had cancer are at equal or increased risk for many chronic diseases as people without the disease, such as other cancers, heart disease, and diabetes. Many factors, such as being physically inactive and overweight, may contribute to these conditions. Although there is little evidence about diet and cancer recurrence, findings continue to suggest a life balance of physical activity, a healthful diet, and a healthful weight as helpful in preventing cancer recurrence. The evidence of a benefit is even stronger for a beneficial impact on the risk of developing a new cancer and several other noncancerous diseases.

Body Mass Index, or BMI, is a way to evaluate a person's weight to find out if they're at a healthful weight or may weigh too much. However, there are other factors that should be considered when judging how much someone should weigh, so BMI measurements should only be used as a general guide. (You can calculate your BMI using the chart on page 194.)

Almost 65 percent of adults in the United States were overweight or obese (BMI greater than 25) in 2002. In the United States, more than 300,000 deaths each year are associated with obesity. The World Health Organization (WHO) has called obesity a global epidemic.

Being overweight may be related to an increase in cancer recurrence and a decrease in life expectancy. Evidence continues to associate obesity with breast cancer recurrence, and data on obesity affecting the prognosis of people with other cancers is growing as well. Those who have or have had cancer and at risk for other illnesses can take control of their health by incorporating physical activity, eating a variety of fresh vegetables and fruits, and maintaining a healthful weight throughout life.

While you're focusing on a plan to give your body what it needs, don't forget to take into account your enjoyment of life as well as your basic health and nutrition priorities. As you develop your nutrition plan, make sure to:

- Include foods you like. If your ability to eat what you normally do or your food cravings change, don't be afraid to bend the rules of traditional meals and foods. It's okay to eat your usual lunch food at dinner time or your typical breakfast meal at dinner, if those items are what appeal to you at that time.

- Choose food packed with nutrients. When you choose between foods, pick those with the most nutrition according to your needs. Your body depends on crucial nutrients to function properly now more than ever.
- Make physical activity a part of your plan. Take part in activities you enjoy. Being active can increase your appetite, help regulate bowel movements, energize you, and boost your mood.
- Consult your health care team. Your dietitian, doctor, and nurse can all contribute information to your eating plan. Together, you can develop a plan that takes into account your health, your body, your cancer, and your treatment. Your dietitian, nurse, or doctor may suggest increasing the number of servings of specific types of food, avoiding certain foods, or increasing your intake of water, for example.

The best plan for you may change over time. Your dietary needs will be different as you prepare for cancer treatment and as you undergo it, after treatment, and as you maintain your long-term health; your body will need varying amounts of certain nutrients in order to face cancer, treatment, and recovery. Reevaluate your dietary needs as you enter new stages of treatment and recovery.

NUTRITIONAL NEEDS MAY BE DIFFERENT FOR PEOPLE WITH CANCER

A diagnosis of cancer motivates some people to try to positively change their lifestyles. Many people change their eating habits after being diagnosed with cancer, while others take dietary supplements.

But which changes in your diet will benefit your body during treatment? The basics of optimal nutrition for people with cancer may not be what you expect. People going through cancer treatment or after treatment need a lot of energy to stay strong when their bodies are fighting disease. The foods you'll be advised to eat during treatment are designed to help you build strength and withstand the effects of cancer treatment. You'll need to eat fairly regularly even if you don't have a strong appetite. That means that higher calorie, higher protein foods often take top billing, while low-fat, low-calorie foods are discouraged. Other people, such as those being treated for breast cancer, may be more likely to gain weight and will want to work with their health care team to make sure not to take in excess calories.

High-calorie, high-protein foods include milk, cheese, and eggs. If you lose weight, your dietitian or health care provider may advise you to eat more sauces and gravies and to include more butter, margarine, or oil in your foods to boost

Analyze Your Diet

Talk to your dietitian about using recipe or nutrient analysis computer programs to track your intake of nutrients if you're concerned about getting enough or are curious about whether or not your meals are balanced. These programs may even track trace minerals and amino acids, calculate recommended daily intakes, and show your eating and nutrient patterns over time.

Many are available free to download from the Internet or can be purchased at a store that carries computer programs. One option is the Interactive Healthy Eating Index from the U.S. Department of Agriculture's Center for Policy and Promotion (*http://147.208.9.133/ Default.asp*). You input the types and amounts of food you eat, and the site evaluates the nutrients in your diet.

Nutrient analysis programs are generally not specific enough to provide in-depth evaluations of the quality of your food, however. They may not differentiate between whole-grain flour and the white flour in a doughnut, for example. The Healthy Eating Index is being reworked to provide more information about diet quality.

calories. Because fiber can aggravate problems such as diarrhea, you may also be encouraged to eat fewer high-fiber foods. Increasing calories and protein without relying on refined sugar, refined starches, and high carbohydrates is the healthiest approach.

Keep Moving

A number of studies have considered the benefit of exercise during cancer treatments. Evidence shows that exercise is safe and possible during treatment, and that it can also help control common side effects of treatment (such as fatigue, pain, and nausea), improve physical, emotional, and functional well-being, and improve quality of life.

Studies show that physical inactivity can lead to obesity and increased risk for cancer of several sites of the colon and rectum, prostate, endometrium, breast (among postmenopausal women), and kidney. No large-scale studies have explored the possible effects of exercise on cancer recurrence or cancer survival rates. More research is necessary to determine if exercise during treatment helps, harms, or has no effect.

Being as active as you're physically able to be is a good strategy for people undergoing cancer treatment as well as those who are beyond therapy and focusing on recovery and wellness. In addition to watching your diet, maintaining some level of exercise also can improve your sense of autonomy, which you may feel you have lost since your cancer diagnosis.

Light, regular exercise can improve your appetite, aid in digestion, prevent constipation, help you keep up your energy level and maintain muscle mass, and help you relax and cope with stress. Making an attempt to get out every day and walk—even 100 yards—early in your cancer treatment will help you stay physically active.

The benefits of exercise in improving an overall quality of life are well known. Taking the stairs instead of the elevator, walking to lunch instead of driving, using the hotel gym (for example, if you're traveling for treatment), or standing while talking on the phone are just a few simple ways of changing your routine to raise your level of physical activity.

Issues to keep in mind as you work physical activity into your treatment plan include:

- If you are in bed because of disease and/or treatment, talk to your health care team about physical therapy in bed to keep up your strength and maintain range of motion. Physical activity can help alleviate the fatigue and depression experienced by some people confined to bed.

- Some people in chemotherapy may want to wait until they have finished two cycles of chemotherapy before starting an exercise program because of fatigue. Other people may not have fatigue early in treatment and may therefore be better able to exercise. Talk to your health care team about physical activity and your situation.

- Older people and those with conditions such as arthritis should pay careful attention to balance to prevent a fall. A caregiver or exercise professional may be able to help stabilize those who need assistance.

Over 30 studies have considered exercise and its effects on the body during and after treatment for breast cancer. While few of the studies were large randomized clinical trials (human trials that are considered the standard for study proof), they indicate that physical activity during and after treatment does benefit women with breast cancer, improving physical fitness (endurance, flexibility, and body composition, for example) and self-esteem, and helping to alleviate stress, depression, and fatigue.

15

Don't Forget Physical Activity

Studies have shown that regular physical activity can reduce anxiety and depression, improve mood, boost self-esteem, and reduce symptoms of fatigue, nausea, pain, and diarrhea. These benefits can be gained through participation in moderate physical activity on most, if not all, days of the week. Physical activity can also be a great opportunity to spend time with a friend, spouse, or child. Talk to your health care team about the level of activity that's appropriate for you.

Type of Physical Activity	What's Involved	Examples
General Physical Activity	Muscle movement that uses energy, including exercise and daily activities	Swimming, dancing, mowing the lawn
Aerobic Activity	Improving cardiovascular fitness	Walking the dog, jogging, bicycling, jumping rope
Resistance Training	Strengthening muscles and protecting joints	Lifting weights or using resistance training equipment, push-ups, carrying, and lifting
Flexibility Training	Stretching muscles to improve range of motion, balance, and stability	Stretching and yoga

Talk to the Experts

No food or diet can cure cancer, although some of them may help with side effects or help your body mend after cancer treatment. Some foods and nutritional choices may help cancer treatment work more effectively or may help keep you healthy. Others can be dangerous and can interfere with treatment and recovery. In the course of your treatment, you may hear about both. How can you tell which will help you eat healthfully and stay healthy before, during, or after treatment?

Along with your doctor or nurse, a registered dietitian is one of your best sources of information about your diet and can add to the information in this

16

book. A registered dietitian is an expert in food and diet, has at least a bachelor's degree, and has passed a national competency exam. (There are no educational requirements associated with the title of nutritionist.) The members of your health care team can provide nutrition help or advice when you need it. For more information or for a referral to a registered dietitian, contact the American Dietetic Association (ADA; 800-366-1655; *http://www.eatright.org*). The ADA helps people locate local registered dietitians, including dietitians specializing in oncology nutrition. The ADA web site contains information on diet and nutrition and a registered dietitian locator service.

If you have a question about something in this book and how it relates to you, your cancer, and your treatment, your health care team can give you more detailed information. You may want to take these steps before asking your health care team about a nutrition topic to ensure that you have a productive conversation:

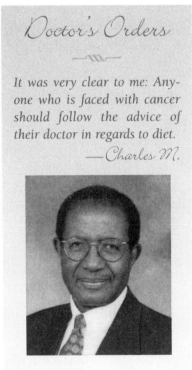

Doctor's Orders

—◆◆◆—

It was very clear to me: Anyone who is faced with cancer should follow the advice of their doctor in regards to diet.

—*Charles M.*

- ❧ Do your own research before appointments and gather information from unbiased and trustworthy information sources. The most reliable sources are often voluntary health organizations; accredited cancer centers; medical, nursing, and dietitians' professional organizations; and government agencies— such as those listed in the *Resources* section of this book.
- ❧ Write down a list of questions.
- ❧ Bring relevant information to appointments. Be sure to note the source of your information so your medical team can determine its reliability.
- ❧ Explain why you want to know about certain topics.
- ❧ Ask a friend or family member to accompany you to appointments to help make sure that your questions are clear and that you get complete answers.

Reliable Research

Be careful to get the facts before pinning hopes on a nutritional strategy. Getting solid information and consulting your health care team can help you determine whether or not a food, supplement, or diet regimen may help or harm your health. When you're looking into something that sounds promising, consider whether or not its claims are likely to hold water by keeping in mind the research strategies that follow.

UNDERSTAND STUDY TYPES

Scientific discoveries are the result of experiments and studies. But some studies are more comprehensive and respected than others. Understanding different types of studies may help you better evaluate their implications.

Laboratory studies. Laboratory studies, or test tube studies, are often the first step in cancer research. Researchers first test substances on bacteria, animal, or human cells grown in laboratory dishes or test tubes. Animal studies may then help researchers learn more about a substance's effects on a whole organism in a controlled environment.

Human studies. Epidemiologic studies look into what influences the way diseases occur in human populations. The two general categories of epidemiologic studies are observational studies and interventional studies:

- Observational studies follow real people going about their normal lives, without any intervention from researchers. In an observational study, researchers studying nutrition and cancer might ask people questions about their diets and look for associations with their cancer prognoses, for example.

- In interventional studies, researchers intentionally change at least one factor they believe is related to the risk of a disease. For example, researchers might suggest that study participants eat a specified amount of certain foods (which could be higher or lower than their usual consumption) or take certain dietary supplements. Then researchers might look for potential effects on cancer risk, prognosis, or recurrence.

  Randomized controlled clinical trials are intervention studies in which people are randomly assigned to one group or another and a factor is intentionally kept different between the two. Randomized controlled clinical trials are the standard for study proof, but they are often difficult to run because of ethical concerns or cost.

STUDY THE CLAIMS

A "breakthrough," "cure for all cancers," or "miracle cure" probably hasn't followed traditional routes of testing and safety. Promises of "miracle cures" or wonder drugs that provide a quick fix are a red flag. Your body and its processes are intricate, and cancer, a group of over 100 diseases, doesn't have one cause or treatment. As you evaluate a product or diet, consider the claims made for the treatment—to cure cancer? to enable the evidence-based treatment to work better? or to relieve symptoms or side effects?

GET THE BACK STORY

News reports often don't have enough space or time to delve into the background details of the promising studies they may report. Simplified versions of the facts may sound more definitive than the evidence actually is. Scientific progress should show a consensus in study results; one study with results out of the norm could be flawed and not indicative of typical effects. Some important information to find out about a study:

- Who conducted the study?
- What type of study was it? Animal studies are conducted early on and aren't always relevant to humans, while human studies are more likely to prove or disprove relevance.
- Who sponsored the study?
- How long did the study last? How large was it? Generally, studies affecting medical policy or guidelines are the result of years of research examining a large number of people.
- Do other studies back up the findings? It usually takes a number of studies with similar results before results are considered definitive.

READ CAREFULLY

Products or diets that count on users' testimonials to prove their effectiveness aren't likely to be based on scientific evidence. Before a promising discovery is translated into medications or other ways of helping people, it should be thoroughly tested and evaluated. Scientific data collected over a period of time and published in a respected, peer-reviewed journal often signals a trustworthy idea. You may want to ask yourself:

- What are the credentials of those supporting the treatment? Are they recognized experts in cancer treatment? Have they published their findings in peer-reviewed, respected journals?
- Is the product or method widely available for use within the health-care community, or is it controlled and access to its use limited?
- Is the product or treatment promoted for use in place of standard therapies or clinical trials?

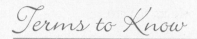

Terms to Know

You may have heard the terms "alternative" or "complementary" used to refer to methods of diagnosing, preventing, or treating cancer and wondered exactly what they meant. How can you know if these approaches are safe and if they are likely to help you? The definitions below can help you sort out what these terms mean.

Proven treatment refers to evidence-based, medical treatments that have been tested following a strict set of guidelines and found to be safe and effective. The results of such studies have been published in peer reviewed journals—that is, journals reviewed by other doctors or scientists in the field. The treatments have been approved by the FDA and are accepted as "mainstream" medicine.

Research or investigational treatments are therapies being studied in a clinical trial. Clinical trials are research projects that determine whether a new treatment is effective and safe for humans. Before a drug or other treatment can be used regularly to treat people, it is studied and tested carefully, first in laboratory test tubes, and then in animals. After these studies are completed and the therapy is found safe and promising, it is tested to see if it helps people who are ill. If this careful testing shows that the drug or other treatment is safe and effective, the FDA may approve it for regular use. Only then does the treatment become part of the standard, mainstream collection of proven therapies used to treat disease in human beings.

Complementary refers to supportive methods that are used to complement, or add to, proven treatments. Examples might include meditation to reduce stress or peppermint tea for nausea. Complementary methods are not given to cure disease, rather they may help control symptoms and improve well-being. Some of the methods, such as massage therapy, yoga, and meditation, that are categorized as complementary have been referred to as supportive care in the past.

The term unproven or untested can be confusing because it is sometimes used to refer to treatments with little basis in scientific fact, while it may also refer to treatments or tests that are under investigation. Adequate scientific evidence is not available to support its use.

Alternative refers to treatments that are promoted as cancer cures. They are unproven because they have not been scientifically tested, or were tested and found to be ineffective. If you use alternative therapies *instead of* evidence-based treatment, you may suffer, either from lack of helpful treatment or because the alternative treatment is harmful.

- Is the treatment or drug a "secret" that only certain providers can give?
- Does the treatment require you to travel to another country?

TURN TO TRUSTWORTHY SOURCES

Snippets of information about cancer and its treatment on the radio, TV, in the newspaper, in magazines, and on the Internet can be both exciting and confusing. Respected health information sources collect, assess, and share established information and can help you tell the difference between preliminary or unfounded findings and established developments you might want to pursue. Keep in mind that evidence-based methods will be promoted in scientific journals and not only in the mass media (books, magazines, TV and radio talk shows). The sources in the *Resources* section in the back of this book are a good place to start your research.

Chapter 2

Foods of Special Interest: Vegetables, Fruits, and Whole Grains

MANY HEALTHFUL COMPOUNDS ARE FOUND in vegetables, fruits, and whole grains, and these compounds most likely work in combination to exert their beneficial effect. There are important, as yet unidentified, components of whole food and synergies with other foods that are not available in supplements. The anticancer effects of any single food cannot be completely understood without evaluating the food as part of a bigger dietary picture. The glucosinolates (a type of phytonutrient) in broccoli, for example, appear to have no benefit of their own. It is still unclear whether it is broccoli's vitamin C, beta-carotene, folate, or other compounds that, working together and in the right quantities, protect individuals against cancer development and improve the health of a person who has cancer.

Rather than relying on one particular food in large amounts, aim for a balanced diet that includes five or more servings a day of a variety of vegetables and fruits, along with foods from a variety of other plant sources, such as whole-grain breads and cereals, nuts, seeds, rice, pasta, and beans.

The way foods affect the body—and especially how they affect the body of a person with an illness like cancer—is complex. It is very difficult to establish the exact role of a particular food in the cancer process. It is even more difficult when the food in question is typically consumed in small amounts. In this chapter we'll go over the basics: what each fruit, vegetable, or grain contains that has the power to help or harm, what's been proven and what is not scientifically

Raw vs. Cooked Produce: The Nutrient Debate

Fresh produce is *usually* considered to have more nutritional value than cooked. Generally, the less produce is cooked, the more nutrients it retains. Boiling vegetables, especially for long periods, can leach out their B and C vitamins. Microwaving and steaming may be the best ways to preserve the nutritional content of vegetables.

However, frozen foods may be more nutritious than fresh foods because they are often picked ripe and quickly frozen. Canning is more likely to reduce the heat-sensitive and water-soluble nutrients (nutrients your body doesn't store and must obtain each day, such as vitamin C and B vitamins) because of the high heat involved in processing. (Be aware that some fruits are packed in heavy syrup and some canned vegetables are high in sodium.)

But don't let conflicting or confusing information keep vegetables and fruits off your plate. Choosing at least five vegetables and fruits a day (not counting potatoes and French fries)—in a variety of forms—is the best way to get the nutrients you need.

determined, and how to evaluate the role of these foods in a balanced diet. We'll continue this discussion in chapter 3.

In some cases, evidence about a food's effects is limited to results from animal studies. Animal studies are very early-stage examinations of a food, and controlled clinical studies in humans are needed to determine the usefulness of foods in cancer treatment and prevention.

Vegetables and Fruits

The majority of beneficial nutrients in produce are more concentrated in vegetables than in fruit. Many vegetables and fruits are excellent sources of vitamins and provide ample fiber (the part of plant foods that the body cannot digest and that helps to move food waste out of the body quickly). Vegetables and fruits also contain other beneficial phytochemicals (also called phytomedicinals, compounds in fruits, vegetables, beans, grains, and other plants that seem to benefit the body and may even fight cancer).

In the majority of population studies, eating more vegetables, fruits, or both has been associated with a lower risk of lung, oral, esophageal, and colon cancer.

A diet high in vegetables and fruits might therefore also help improve cancer survival, but there have been few studies of this relationship in people with cancer. However, as outlined in chapter 1, it's a sensible idea for most people with cancer to follow the general dietary recommendations issued by the ACS and many other public health and medical organizations for eating five servings or more of vegetables and fruits a day.

Broccoli (and Other Cruciferous Vegetables)

Broccoli is a cruciferous vegetable (a plant that often has four flowers resembling a cross) that belongs to the cabbage and mustard families, which also includes arugula, cauliflower, collards, bok choy, kale, mustard greens, radishes, turnips, watercress, rutabaga, and brussels sprouts.

Raw broccoli may have a slightly bitter taste. (Cooking broccoli reduces the bitterness.) Ironically, the bitter taste can be traced to the same chemicals thought to provide cancer protection. As a result, scientists have developed different types of broccoli, such as broccolini, a cross between broccoli and Chinese kale, which looks like asparagus and tastes sweeter than broccoli.

Broccoli contains certain chemicals that may reduce the risk of cancer—colorectal cancer in particular—although it is not clear which individual compounds are responsible for the protective effects. Broccoli is considered one of the best sources of nutrients because it is rich in vitamin C, beta-carotene, fiber, calcium, and folate. It is the source of many phytochemicals, which are thought to stimulate the production of anti-cancer enzymes and chemicals. The chemical composition of cruciferous vegetables is complex, which makes it difficult to determine which compound or combination of compounds may provide protection against cancer. Eating a wide variety of plant-based foods is the best way to get the necessary components.

WHAT IS THE EVIDENCE?
Studies have shown that the frequent consumption of cruciferous vegetables as part of a well-rounded healthy diet is associated with a decreased risk for cancer of the colon and bladder. Randomized clinical trials are needed to determine the exact nature of the association.

ARE THERE ANY POSSIBLE PROBLEMS OR COMPLICATIONS?
Since broccoli is a food high in fiber, eating large amounts of it may cause gas. People with diarrhea should avoid or reduce their intake of high-fiber foods.

Phytochemical Power

The term phytochemicals refers to a wide variety of compounds produced by plants. They are found in fruits, vegetables, beans, grains, and other plants. Scientists have identified thousands of phytochemicals. Some of the more commonly known phytochemicals include beta-carotene, ascorbic acid (vitamin C), folic acid, and vitamin E.

Eating vegetables, fruits, and grains reduces cancer risk. Some scientists estimate that people can reduce their risk of cancer by 30 to 40 percent simply by eating more vegetables, fruits, and other plant sources that contain phytochemicals. Researchers are looking for specific compounds in these foods that may account for the beneficial effects in humans.

There is some evidence that phytochemicals may help prevent the formation of potential cancer-causing substances, block the action of carcinogens on their target organs or tissue, or act on cells to suppress cancer development.

Phytochemicals (also called phytomedicinals) are present in all of the vegetables, fruits, legumes (beans and peas), and grains we eat, so it is easy for most people to include them in their diet. For instance, a carrot contains more than 100 phytochemicals. According to one estimate, more than 4,000 phytochemicals are catalogued, but only about 150 have been studied in detail. The information below outlines a few of the phytochemicals researchers have studied.

There is no evidence that taking phytochemical supplements is as beneficial as consuming the vegetables, fruits, beans, and grains from which they are taken. (See chapter 5 for more information about supplements.) Hundreds of phytochemicals in plants play roles in keeping us healthy.

Polyphenols, Flavonoids, and Phytoestrogens
There are several major groups of phytochemicals. One group, the polyphenols, includes a subgroup of chemicals called flavonoids. These plant chemicals are found in a range of grains, vegetables, and fruits. The flavonoids found in soybeans, soy products, garbanzo beans, chickpeas, licorice, and tea may mimic the actions of estrogen (a female sex hormone linked to the growth of some cancers, such as breast cancer). Estrogen-like substances from these plant sources are called phytoestrogens. (Most phytoestrogens are relatively weak and are present in foods in small amounts. Not all flavonoids are phytoestrogens.) Flavonoids are being studied to determine whether they can prevent chronic diseases such as cancer and heart disease.

Antioxidants
Antioxidants make up another category of phytochemicals. Antioxidants protect the body's cells against free radicals (by-products of the body's normal processes), which can damage a cell's DNA and are thought to trigger some forms of cancer and other diseases.

Antioxidants, such as vitamin C, vitamin E, beta-carotene, and lycopene, are found in vegetables such as broccoli, brussels sprouts, cabbage, and cauliflower as well as tomatoes, corn, carrots, mangos, sweet potatoes, soybeans, cantaloupe, oranges, spinach, nuts, lettuce, celery, liver, fish oil, seeds, grains, and black and green tea. While all fruits and vegetables are beneficial to the body, eating a variety of dark-colored vegetables and fruits, which contain higher levels of antioxidants and other phytochemicals than other vegetables and fruits, is a good way to take in more antioxidants.

Carotenoids and Anthocyanins

Carotenoids, which give carrots, yams, cantaloupe, butternut squash, and apricots their orange color, are also promoted as anticancer agents. Tomatoes, red peppers, and red grapefruit contain lycopene, which is a powerful antioxidant (see the *Tomatoes* section on page 28 of this chapter for more information about lycopene).

The phytochemicals lutein and zeaxanthin, found in spinach, kale, and turnip greens, may reduce the risk of lung cancer. According to some nutritionists, grapes, eggplant, red cabbage, and radishes all contain anthocyanins—phytochemicals that protect against cancer and heart disease. Ellagic acid, found in raspberries, blackberries, cranberries, strawberries, and walnuts, also is said to have anticancer effects.

Sulfides

Another group of phytochemicals called sulfides are found in garlic and onions. Sulfides may reduce the risk of stomach cancer, lower blood pressure, and strengthen the immune system. (See the *Garlic* section on page 38 of chapter 3 for more information about sulfides.)

Much of the evidence about phytochemicals' powerful effects so far has come from observations of cultures whose diets consist mainly of plant sources, and which appear to experience noticeably lower rates of certain types of cancer and heart disease. Some of the associations between individual phytochemicals and cancer risk are very compelling and make a very strong case for additional investigation. To date, none of the findings are conclusive, and knowledge about which of the numerous phytochemicals in vegetables and fruits actively help the body fight disease remains to be determined.

Until conclusive research findings emerge, health care professionals advise a balanced diet with emphasis on a wide variety of vegetables, fruits, legumes, and whole grains.

Mushrooms

Shiitake mushrooms, edible fungi native to Asia and grown in forests, are the second most commonly cultivated edible mushrooms in the world.

Promoters claim that eating the whole shiitake mushroom (cap and stem) may have therapeutic value, but they do not say how much must be eaten to have an effect. Natural shiitake mushrooms are widely available in grocery stores.

WHAT IS THE EVIDENCE?
There is no current evidence that eating mushrooms fights cancer in humans.

ARE THERE ANY POSSIBLE PROBLEMS OR COMPLICATIONS?
Shiitake mushrooms are generally considered safe. No adverse reactions have been reported when eaten at normal doses, with the exception of people with allergies to mushrooms.

Tomatoes

Lycopene is the compound that gives tomatoes and certain other vegetables and fruits their color. It is one of the major carotenoids in the diet of North Americans. (See the *Phytochemical Power* section in this chapter for more information about carotenoids and other phytochemicals.)

Dietary lycopene comes primarily from tomatoes, although apricots, guava, watermelon, papaya, and pink grapefruit are also significant sources. Tomato products are the best source of lycopene; initial studies have suggested that processed tomatoes eaten along with oil or fat (in tomato sauce or paste, for example) are a more readily absorbed source of available lycopene than raw tomato juice. The heating action evaporates much of the water, leaving the more easily absorbed pulp that contains the lycopene. Also, since lycopene is a fat-soluble nutrient, the oil found in tomato sauces is thought to help promote its absorption.

Vegetables for Health

——

Sweet potatoes and pumpkin are both excellent sources of beta-carotene, easy to prepare, and easily digested.
— *Norma Jean*

I eat vegetables with dinner every night and cereal in the morning with a multivitamin/mineral supplement to make sure I get the nutrients my body needs.
— *Paulette*

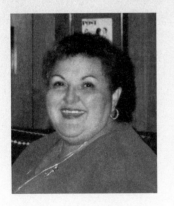

28

It's All in the Label

How can you determine the nutritional value of vegetables and fruits? Simply look at the Nutrition Facts panel on the side or back of labels of frozen and canned items. Nutrition information also is available for many fresh items under the Food and Drug Administration's (FDA's) voluntary point-of-purchase nutrition information program for raw foods. This information may appear on the labels of packaged fresh vegetables and fruits or on posters or brochures in the produce area.

The nutrition information lists the kinds and amounts of important nutrients in a serving of the fruit or vegetable and gives the Percent Daily Value, which shows how much those amounts contribute to the daily diet.

Some information is required: for example, the amount of fat, fiber, vitamins A and C, and iron and calcium, even if there is none. Some labels will carry additional information, such as the amount of folic acid and iron, depending on the types of label claims made.

You can quickly find vegetables and fruits that provide the nutrients you're looking for— for example, vitamin A or C or both—by looking for short descriptive terms on the front, side or back of the food label. For example, an orange juice label may say "provides 100 percent of the Daily Value for vitamin C." These claims refer to the contents of one serving of the item.

Less frequently, you may see longer claims describing the relationship between the labeled food or one or more nutrients in the food to a certain disease or medical condition. Only claims approved by the FDA can be used in food labeling. Three approved health claims pertain to vegetables and fruits. These claims can describe how:

- vegetables and fruits may help lower the risk of some cancers
- fruits, vegetables, and grain products that contain fiber, particularly soluble fiber, may help reduce the risk of coronary heart disease
- fiber-containing grain products, vegetables, and fruits may help reduce the risk of some cancers

In addition, in spring 1996, the FDA approved a claim stating that a diet with adequate folic acid may reduce the risk of certain birth defects. This claim might appear, for example, on labels of dried beans, brussels sprouts, asparagus, tomato juice, and orange juice—foods that are excellent or good sources of folate.

Food labeling of fresh, frozen, and canned vegetables and fruits may carry the message, too. And if you need more specific nutrition information about a particular item, you can find it in the labeling of most products, as well. The FDA regulates this information.

Berry Good

Researchers have discovered that cranberries, blackcurrants, lingonberries (related to cranberries), and bilberries (which are like blueberries) contain high levels of a flavonoid called quercetin that may fight cancer. Onions, green beans, lettuce, and rhubarb (as well as red wine) are other sources of quercetin.

In the lab, quercetin is a powerful antioxidant. A recent study involving forty 60-year-old men had them eat either 100 grams (approximately ⅕ pound, or 3½ ounces) a day of blackcurrants, lingonberries, and bilberries for eight weeks or eat their normal diets. The men eating the berries saw their blood quercetin levels increase 30 to 50 percent compared to the other men.

Berries also contain fiber, vitamin C, other flavonoids, and other compounds that may inhibit the growth of certain types of human tumors. Many of the antioxidants in berries are destroyed when they are cooked or frozen.

People who frequently incorporate tomatoes into their diet appear to have a lower risk of certain types of cancer, especially cancers of the prostate, lung, and stomach. Further research is needed to determine what role, if any, lycopene has in the prevention or treatment of cancer.

Some researchers believe lycopene may be valuable in the prevention of cancer as well as stopping the growth of cancers of the prostate, lung, and stomach. These scientists note that lycopene is a powerful antioxidant, a compound that blocks the action of activated oxygen molecules, known as free radicals, which can damage cells.

The antioxidant activity of lycopene is at least twice as great as beta-carotene, another carotenoid that is also thought to be an effective cancer-preventing nutrient. (See the Vitamin A information in chapter 5 for more information about beta-carotene.)

WHAT IS THE EVIDENCE?

Studies suggest that diets rich in tomato intake are associated with a lower risk of several different types of cancer. The strongest evidence is for a protective effect against cancers of the lung, stomach, and prostate gland. There may also be a protective benefit against cancers of the cervix, breast, oral cavity, pancreas, colon, rectum, and esophagus. However, a direct relationship with these cancers has not yet been proven. Other compounds in tomatoes or in those diets high in tomato products, either acting alone or with lycopene, may be responsible for the protective effects currently associated with lycopene.

ARE THERE ANY POSSIBLE PROBLEMS OR COMPLICATIONS?
Lycopene obtained from eating vegetables and fruits has no known side effects and is safe for humans.

Whole Grains

The complex carbohydrates in grain foods provide the body with energy. The indigestible fiber and phytochemicals in whole grains make them a useful cancer-fighting food. But in the United States, people eat on average only half a serving of whole grains a day, which means we miss out on much of the folate, selenium, and other nutrients in whole grains. Brown rice, millet, quinoa, kasha (buckwheat), barley, whole-wheat pasta, and bulgur are good sources of whole grains. Between 15 and 20 percent of cereals contain whole grain as a main ingredient.

A whole grain contains the germ (the sprout of a new plant), endosperm (the seed's source of energy), and bran (the outer layer) of a grain or seed. Refined grains such as bleached flour have the bran and germ removed during milling and therefore lack many of the nutrients found in whole grains, including B vitamins, iron, zinc, phytochemicals, vitamin E, and fiber.

Dietary fiber includes a wide variety of plant carbohydrates that are not digested by humans. Specific categories of fiber are soluble (dissolvable in water), such as oat bran, or insoluble (not dissolvable in water), such as wheat bran or cellulose. (Soluble fiber helps to reduce blood cholesterol, thereby lowering the risk of coronary heart disease.) Good sources of fiber are beans, vegetables, whole grains, and fruits.

Associations between the fiber in whole grains and cancer risk are inconclusive, but eating these foods is still recommended because they contain other substances that can help prevent cancer and because they have other health benefits. Fiber is best obtained from whole grains, vegetables, and fruits.

Since whole grains are high in fiber, eating large amounts of them may cause gas. People with diarrhea should avoid or reduce their intake of high-fiber foods.

Whole-Grain Benefits

Many of the carbohydrates eaten in the United States (like sugars and refined starches) don't do the body much good. On the other side of the carbohydrate spectrum are whole grains, which vary in nutritional content but contain many more nutrients than refined grains.

Why you should eat more whole grains:

- To help maintain a healthy body and weight. Eating plenty of fiber-containing foods such as whole grains (and also many vegetables and fruits) promotes proper bowel function. The high fiber content of many whole grains may also help you to feel full with fewer calories.
- To live a longer life. A study of 35,000 women showed that those who ate at least one serving of whole grains a day lived longer than women who ate few or no whole grains.
- To protect against cancer. Many studies show the effect of eating whole grains on lowering cancer risk. Their phytochemicals stop damage to DNA and protect against cancer growth.

Ways to eat more whole grains:

- Eat whole-grain bread instead of white, and choose oatmeal over a bagel or English muffin.
- Add whole grains like barley to your soup instead of noodles, and opt for whole-wheat pasta over other noodles.
- Try whole-wheat crackers as a snack.
- Choose whole-wheat flour over refined white flour. (Because it contains the wheat germ and higher fiber, nutritional, and fat content, it should be stored in the refrigerator to prevent spoilage.)
- Experiment with bulgur, millet, quinoa, and pearl barley.

How to spot whole-grain foods:

- Dark breads aren't necessarily whole grain. They may be made with refined white flour and added darkening agents like molasses.
- Look for unprocessed foods and foods with whole grains listed *as the first ingredient* on the Nutrition Facts panel. "Multigrain," "Seven Grain," and "Made with Whole Grain" labels don't mean a food is whole grain. Only whole-grain foods may be labeled as "Whole Grain."

- The Nutrition Facts panel will show you how much fiber a food contains. Two grams or more of fiber per serving qualifies a food as whole grain.
- A claim can be made that a food is a "good source" of fiber if it provides ten percent (2½ grams) of the Daily Value (25 grams) of fiber per serving. Foods can be called "high in fiber," "rich in fiber," or "excellent source of fiber" if they contain 20 percent (five grams) of the Daily Value of fiber per serving.
- "100 percent Whole-Grain" foods or foods with the claim "Diets rich in whole grain foods and other plant foods low in total fat, saturated fat, and cholesterol may reduce the risk of heart disease and certain cancers" (which contain 51 percent or more whole-grain ingredients by weight) are whole-grain foods.

Carbohydrates and the Glycemic Index

All carbohydrates, including complex carbohydrates (vegetables, nuts, seeds, legumes, and whole grains), simple carbohydrates (bread, pasta, and other starches), and sugars (table sugar, honey, and candy), are broken down into sugar in the intestines when they are digested. This sugar enters the blood and raises blood sugar levels. The body reacts by producing more insulin, which helps the body's cells get energy from sugar. This typically regulates blood sugar levels.

The glycemic index is one way of classifying foods. It measures how quickly and how high a person's blood sugar level rises after eating a food. High-glycemic foods cause fast, significant increases in a person's blood sugar levels. Highly processed carbohydrates, in which the bran and germ layers are removed, are high glycemic (they make blood sugar levels shoot higher). Grains that aren't processed as much are absorbed more slowly—which means that whole-grain items are generally low glycemic. (Any proteins and fats you eat along with carbohydrates also affect the speed at which carbohydrates enter the bloodstream and raise insulin levels.)

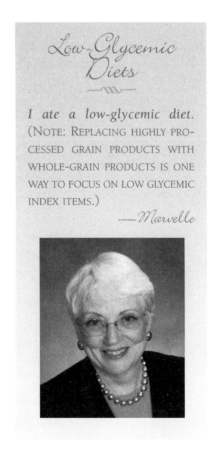

Low-Glycemic Diets

I ate a low-glycemic diet. (NOTE: REPLACING HIGHLY PROCESSED GRAIN PRODUCTS WITH WHOLE-GRAIN PRODUCTS IS ONE WAY TO FOCUS ON LOW GLYCEMIC INDEX ITEMS.)

—Marvelle

High-glycemic foods include refined or simple carbohydrates and are processed by the body quickly, rapidly raising blood levels:

- potatoes
- white rice
- white bread
- pasta (not whole wheat)
- bananas
- sweetened soft drinks and juices
- refined flour products
- sugar and other natural sweeteners

Low-glycemic foods contain unrefined or complex carbohydrates, take longer to digest, and raise blood levels more slowly:

- whole grains (whole wheat, rye, oats, and bran)
- brown rice
- couscous
- quinoa
- barley
- bulgur
- beans and most other legumes
- many whole fruits
- 100 percent whole-grain breakfast cereal

Choosing less-processed whole grains over highly processed products is one simple way to eat for health. Many health professionals recommend eating fewer refined and simple sugars and selecting low-glycemic carbohydrates along with a variety of healthy proteins and fats to balance your daily intake of foods.

Chapter 3

Other Foods of Special Interest

Certain foods are purported to cause cancer, prevent it, help the fight against cancer and recurrence, or hinder it. The foods addressed in this chapter are those that are most often asked about by people with cancer. Some are recognized for having protective properties, others for their potential aid during cancer treatment, and still others have not been proven to have any effect or are considered harmful to healthy people, people with cancer, or people undergoing cancer treatment, and should be avoided.

For the purposes of this chapter, we will consider "foods" substances you consume in the forms in which they are typically sold through grocery stores (for example, soy foods can be found as soybeans, soy milk, tofu, and other forms; green tea is the liquid from brewed, dried tea leaves). However, some of the substances in the foods discussed here are also available in supplement form. (The substances in supplements are often more concentrated than they are when naturally occurring in foods; therefore supplements may cause different effects on the body than eating moderate amounts of the foods themselves as part of a balanced diet. Food sources naturally contain a variety of healthful ingredients that may act together to affect cancer risk; supplements do not. For more information about supplements, see chapter 5.)

Keep in mind that rather than relying on one particular food, even if it may have beneficial health effects, is not a sound nutritional strategy. Eating a varied diet of foods in moderation—including five or more servings a day of vegetables and fruits along with a variety of breads, cereals, grain products, rice, pasta, and beans—is the best way to eat healthfully before, during, and after cancer treatment.

Other Foods of Special Interest to People with Cancer

In the last chapter, we discussed the role of whole grains and various fruits and vegetables in a healthy, balanced diet. We emphasized that the way foods affect the body is complex, and that it is difficult to determine the exact role of a particular food in fighting cancer. Continue to keep this in mind as we look at some additional foods of special interest in this chapter

Coffee

Coffee contains caffeine, a mild stimulant also found in soft drinks and tea.

WHAT IS THE EVIDENCE?

Caffeine may heighten symptoms of fibrocystic breast lumps (a type of benign breast disease) in some women, but no evidence has shown that it increases the risk of breast cancer or other types of cancer.

Although several large-scale studies have been conducted to determine whether there is an association between coffee intake and cancer risk, most of them have not found an increased incidence of cancer among people who drink coffee.

The possible link between coffee and cancer of the pancreas, widely publicized in the past, is controversial and has not been confirmed by other studies. Most studies have shown no substantial association, and evidence indicates that coffee is not significantly related to pancreatic cancer risk.

ARE THERE ANY POSSIBLE PROBLEMS OR COMPLICATIONS?

Drinking coffee in moderation does not promote the growth of cancer cells.

The caffeine in coffee has a diuretic effect on the body that lasts for a couple of hours after it is consumed, so drinking many cups of coffee may contribute to dehydration.

Does Sugar Feed Cancer Cells?

Some people believe that cancer thrives off of sugar and recommend that people with cancer stop eating sugar. Because individuals who consume large amounts of sugar generally do not eat adequate amounts of cancer-protective vegetables and fruits and consume more fatty meats, factors besides sugar intake may account for any increase in cancer risk.

Highly-refined or highly-sugared foods, which are low in nutrients, low in fiber, and high in carbohydrates, contribute calories to the diet but little else. Foods high in refined sugars or carbohydrates may also increase insulin resistance (see the *Carbohydrates and the Glycemic Index* section on page 33 of chapter 2). It isn't known whether this is important in cancer survival, but it is likely to factor into increasing obesity and to increase the risk of diabetes and cardiovascular disease. There is increasing interest in the possibility that refined carbohydrates and sugared foods may increase the risk of certain cancers such as breast, colorectal, or pancreatic cancer.

Taking in enough calories and keeping up your energy may be your goal during treatment. Your health care team may advise you to include high-calorie foods in your diet in order to meet this goal. Including refined carbohydrates or sugared foods in your diet will help you maintain weight if you are losing more than you should. While a healthful diet before and after treatment may include these foods in moderation, it's a good idea to avoid large amounts of sugar, since it contains only calories and no nutritional value. Emphasize a well-balanced selection of foods, including complex carbohydrates, proteins, and fats. *Sugar does not cause cancer, nor, despite the claims of some "alternative" practitioners, does it hasten the growth of cancer cells.*

Flaxseed

Flaxseed—also called linseed—has been promoted since the 1950s as a dietary nutrient with anticancer properties. Flaxseed is available in flour, meal, and seed form and is found in some multi-grain breads, cereals, breakfast bars, and muffins. The toasted seeds are sometimes mixed into bread dough or sprinkled over salads, yogurt, or cereal. Since the substances in flaxseeds are concentrated in flaxseed oil, the potential for side effects is greater when the oil is used. Ground flaxseeds can be stored in the freezer where they won't spoil.

The flaxseed is a rich source of lignans, compounds that can act as anti-estrogens or as weak estrogens (female hormones) and may play a role in preventing estrogen-dependent cancers such as breast cancer and other cancers. Lignans may also function as antioxidants and may slow cell growth in ways not yet understood.

WHAT IS THE EVIDENCE?
Most of the evidence of flaxseed's ability to prevent cancer from occurring or growing has come from a few studies in animals. Randomized clinical trials are needed to study flaxseed's effects on cancer.

ARE THERE ANY POSSIBLE PROBLEMS OR COMPLICATIONS?
Some possible side effects include diarrhea, gas, and nausea. Flaxseed oil should not be used with other laxatives or stool softeners.

Garlic

Garlic (*Allium sativum*) is a member of the lily family and is closely related to onions, leeks, shallots, scallions, and chives. Proponents claim that garlic has anticancer properties as well as antibacterial and medicinal properties that may help stomach and abdominal problems.

There is considerable debate as to how the form and amount of garlic used might influence health. Because processing the garlic clove, including cooking, reduces the activity of its active ingredients, it may be best to mince and eat it raw.

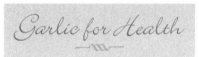

Garlic for Health

I ate garlic regularly as a healthful antioxidant, but the changes in my sense of taste made garlic virtually indiscernible as a flavor to me. I'm sure this wasn't much appreciated by my caregivers at times.

— *Kathi*

WHAT IS THE EVIDENCE?
Garlic may reduce the levels of *Helicobacter pylori*, a bacteria found in the stomach of infected individuals. This bacteria has been linked with stomach cancer.

ARE THERE ANY POSSIBLE PROBLEMS OR COMPLICATIONS?
Consumption of large amounts of garlic may lead to irritation of the gastrointestinal tract, causing stomach pain, gas, and vomiting. One study suggests that the use of garlic may increase the risk of bleeding due to its anti–blood clotting properties. It should not be used by people who are undergoing surgery, especially if they have been given blood thinners or if postoperative bleeding is a concern.

Does Eating Salt or Salt-preserved Foods Affect Cancer Risk or Growth?

Many recommendations for a balanced diet include avoiding excess salt. Studies in other countries link diets containing large amounts of foods preserved by salting and pickling with an increased risk of stomach, nasopharyngeal, and throat cancers. Eating meats preserved by methods involving smoke or salt should be reduced to lessen exposure to potential cancer-causing substances, but no evidence suggests that salt used in cooking or in flavoring foods affects cancer risk.

Some proponents claim that a diet high in sodium (salt) and low in potassium promotes tumor growth by changing the normal pH and water balance in human cells. This theory has not been supported by either clinical or experimental data.

More research and scientific scrutiny is needed before any specific recommendations about sodium are made for people with cancer. People with cancer can help maintain a healthful diet by eating salty snacks and salting food in moderation.

Ginger

Ginger is a plant native to southeast Asia that is also grown in the United States, China, India, and various tropical regions. Ginger has a long history as a pungent spice for cooking and has been used to control or prevent nausea, vomiting, and motion sickness; as an anti-inflammatory (a drug that reduces pain and swelling as in arthritis), a cold remedy, and an aid to digestion; and as a remedy for intestinal gas.

WHAT IS THE EVIDENCE?

Ginger tea and other foods that contain real ginger reduce nausea in some, but not all, controlled studies in humans. Studies also show that ginger reduces motion sickness and severe vomiting in pregnancy. Studies of ginger's ability to reduce nausea and vomiting associated with surgery have had mixed results. Ginger may not help combat nausea during chemotherapy because it affects the stomach rather than the central nervous system. Some brands of ginger snaps, ginger ale, and ginger candy contain real ginger (as does tea made from ginger root).

Ginger does not stop tumor growth, regardless of claims made by some who sell it.

ARE THERE ANY POSSIBLE PROBLEMS OR COMPLICATIONS?
The taste and aroma of ginger and ginger-containing foods and beverages may be calming for some individuals. In rare cases, some people have experienced an allergic reaction to ginger and occasional mild upset stomach.

It is generally considered reasonable and safe to drink ginger ale or eating ginger candy made with real ginger in efforts to control nausea. However, consult your doctor before attempting to use ginger to control nausea related to chemotherapy.

Large doses of ginger may interfere with blood clotting and blood-thinning medications such as warfarin (Coumadin).

Green Tea

Green tea is a drink made from the steamed and dried leaves of the *Camellia sinesis* plant, a shrub native to Asia. Black tea is also made from this plant, but unlike green tea, it is made from leaves that have been dried and fermented. (Herbal teas are made from fruit and spices instead of tea leaves. Therefore herbal teas don't contain the antioxidants found in actual teas.)

The Chinese have been drinking green tea to promote good health for at least 3,000 years. Green tea is widely consumed in Japan, China, and other Asian nations and is becoming more popular in Western nations. Although tea is consumed in a variety of ways and varies in its chemical makeup, one study showed steeping green or black tea for about five minutes released over 80 percent of its catechins (antioxidants). (Instant iced tea contains almost no catechins.)

Some researchers believe green tea may have a protective effect against some cancers because it contains chemicals known as polyphenols, which have antioxidant properties. (An antioxidant is a compound that blocks the action of activated oxygen molecules, known as free radicals, which can damage cells.) One major element in green tea is a catechin, a type of antioxidant. This compound is believed to block production of an enzyme required for cancer cell growth. This catechin may work by suppressing the formation of blood vessels, a process called angiogenesis, thereby cutting off the supply of blood to cancer cells.

WHAT IS THE EVIDENCE?

Some reports indicate green tea may have the ability to help prevent certain cancers from developing, including prostate, stomach, and esophageal cancers. However, results from human studies have been mixed. There has been little study of the effects of drinking tea on people with cancer.

ARE THERE ANY POSSIBLE PROBLEMS OR COMPLICATIONS?

Green tea is generally considered safe. A daily cup or two of green tea is not known to be at all harmful. However, some people may develop allergic reactions and should stop drinking it.

If you are taking warfarin (Coumadin) or other blood thinners, do not drink large amounts of green tea. (Drinking large amounts of green tea—a half gallon to a full gallon a day—could reduce the effects of these drugs).

Drinking large amounts of tea may cause nutritional and other problems because of the caffeine content (which in high doses contributes to dehydration) and its tannins, which may reduce the body's absorption of iron (this is similar to how nutrients in spinach bind to iron and make it difficult for the body to absorb it). Individuals with cancer who are having problems with eating and maintaining weight might need to substitute tea for higher calorie liquids.

Omega-3 Fatty Acids (Fish, Fish Oil, and Legumes)

Omega-3 fatty acids are important nutrients involved in many human biological processes. The body cannot make these chemicals and must obtain them from outside sources.

Oils from some cold-water fish—such as sardines, salmon, herring, mackerel, halibut, striped bass, tuna, shark, and cod—have high concentrations of omega-3 fatty acids. (Oil from flaxseed contains more alpha-linolenic acid [one of the three omega-3 fatty acids] than any other known plant source. See the *Flaxseed* section on page 37 of this chapter for more information.) Other plant sources of omega-3 fatty acids include walnuts, Great Northern beans, kidney beans, navy beans, and soybeans.

Some clinicians believe that omega-3 fatty acids protect against the spread of cancers that are related to hormone production, particularly breast cancer, and that they inhibit the growth of colon, pancreatic, and prostate cancers. Omega-3 fatty acids may reduce the physical wasting and malnourishment that can occur during later stages of some cancers.

Some nutritionists recommend eating a diet rich in fish containing omega-3 fatty acids or eating one to two teaspoons of flaxseed daily.

WHAT IS THE EVIDENCE?
Studies in animals have found that fish fats rich in omega-3 fatty acids suppress cancer formation. The evidence from the few studies on humans published in peer-reviewed medical journals is mixed.

ARE THERE ANY POSSIBLE PROBLEMS OR COMPLICATIONS?
Not enough is known about omega-3 fatty acids to determine if they are safe in large quantities or in the presence of other drugs. Omega-3s may increase total blood cholesterol and inhibit blood clotting. People who take anticoagulant drugs or aspirin should not consume additional amounts of omega-3 due to the risk of excessive bleeding.

The source of omega-3 fatty acids may be a health concern. Many fish caught in the wild contain toxic substances absorbed from environmental pollutants. Experts recommend varying the type of fish eaten to reduce the chances of ingesting poisonous contaminated substances. Swordfish and shark, for instance, both of which are high in omega-3 fatty acids, may also contain high levels of mercury. Farm-raised fish tend to carry fewer toxic substances than fish in the wild.

Soy

Soybeans can be consumed in many forms, such as tofu, soybeans (edamame), soy milk, and soy powder. The amount of isoflavones (compounds that act like weak forms of estrogens naturally produced in the body, sometimes called phytoestrogens or plant estrogens) varies between different types of tofu and soy milk products. As a protein source, soybean products are promoted as a healthier protein alternative to eating meat. Genistein and daidzein, both soy isoflavones, are thought to be the main factors responsible for the protective effects of soy. Other active components of soy may also account for the response in individuals who regularly consume soy products.

WHAT IS THE EVIDENCE?
Results of research on the effects of eating isoflavones on cancer risk have been mixed.

42

Alcohol and Cancer

Numerous studies have linked drinking alcohol to the risk for some primary cancers, such as cancers of the head and neck; however, there is not much evidence to link alcohol intake with a risk for cancer recurrence and an effect on survival. In theory, drinking alcohol could influence a person's risk for new primary cancers of the head and neck, pancreas, liver, and breast. Drinking alcohol can raise levels of estrogens in the body which theoretically might promote estrogen-dependent cancers such as breast and endometrial cancers. Talk to your doctor about your situation, potential risk, and any recommendations for limiting your alcohol.

For the population at large, drinking one to two drinks a day (one drink is defined as four ounces of wine, 12 ounces of beer, or one to one and a half ounces of liquor) is associated with a lower risk of heart disease. Some people with cancer will be at risk for heart disease—as well as for cancer recurrence and new primary cancers—so each individual and his or her health care team should consider the potential impact of drinking alcohol on the person's health.

Drinking moderately before meals may benefit someone with cancer by stimulating his or her hunger when experiencing a decreased appetite. However, alcoholic beverages provide calories but not many nutrients. It's especially important for people with cancer to not replace nutrient-rich food with alcohol because they may have increased nutritional needs.

ARE THERE ANY POSSIBLE PROBLEMS OR COMPLICATIONS?

Soy may reduce the effectiveness of tamoxifen, a drug taken for estrogen-receptor positive breast cancer. The isoflavones in soy have weak estrogen-like activity, and it remains uncertain how this affects the growth of estrogen receptor-positive breast cancers. Some researchers suggest they may act as anti-estrogens and reduce cancer growth, while others suggest their estrogenic activity could cause cancers to grow faster. Until this issue is resolved, many oncologists recommend that people who take tamoxifen or people with estrogen-sensitive breast tumors should avoid the addition of large amounts of soy foods to their diets. It is fine to consume soy as part of a balanced diet; because of its potential effects on the body, some cancer dietitians recommend that women with breast cancer limit their intake of soy (dietitians' recommendations may range, for example, from no more than two to three half-cup servings a day to no more than the equivalent of three half-cup servings a week).

The consumption of soybeans is generally considered safe. Side effects are rare, but may include occasional gastrointestinal problems such as stomach pain, loose stool, and diarrhea.

Chapter 4

Food Quality and Safety

A S YOU CONSIDER NUTRITION AND ITS IMPORTANT EFFECTS on cancer and treatment, you may also be thinking about the quality and safety of the food sources you're relying on. You may wonder if pesticides or organic, genetically modified, or irradiated food contribute any complicating factors to the equation.

Food Factors

People with cancer may wonder if the way food is raised or treated might affect their health. In this chapter we'll explain factors related to food quality and safety, why you might have heard about them as issues relevant to people with cancer, and if they might affect you. We discuss food safety and handling in greater detail in chapter 10.

Pesticides

According to the Environmental Protection Agency's (EPA's) Office of Pesticide Programs, a pesticide is any substance or mixture of substances intended to prevent, destroy, repel, or reduce any pest. Pests can be insects, mice, and other animals, unwanted plants (weeds), fungi, or microorganisms like bacteria and viruses. Though often misunderstood as referring only to insecticides, the term pesticide also applies to herbicides (chemicals that kill weeds) and fungicides (chemicals that kill fungi).

Pesticides are applied to many commercially grown fruit and vegetable crops to help protect them from insects, diseases, weeds, and mold. Pesticides are closely regulated by the EPA, the Food and Drug Administration (FDA), and the United States Department of Agriculture (USDA).

ARE PESTICIDES SAFE?

Pesticides play a valuable role in sustaining the food supply. Pesticide residues in the vegetables and fruits you buy or grow pose very little risk to human health. Although vegetables and fruits sometimes contain low levels of pesticides, no evidence shows that residues of pesticides and herbicides at the low doses found in foods increase the risk of cancer or recurrence. The overall health benefits and cancer-protective effects of eating vegetables and fruits are supported by overwhelming scientific evidence. *The benefits of a balanced diet rich in vegetables and fruits far outweigh the largely theoretical risks posed by occasional, very low pesticide residue levels in foods.*

If you are concerned about even minor risks during cancer treatment, using organically grown foods can reduce your exposure to pesticides.

If you're concerned about pesticide residues on non-organic foods, here are some steps you can take to reduce your risk further:

- Wash vegetables and fruits with large amounts of cold or warm tap water and scrub with a dish brush when appropriate—for example, before eating apples, cucumbers, potatoes, or other produce in which the outer skin or peel is consumed. Do not use soap.
- Throw away the outer leaves of leafy vegetables, such as lettuce and cabbage.
- Peel and cook produce when appropriate, although some nutrients and fiber may be lost when produce is peeled and cooked.

Genetically Modified Foods

Genetically modified (GM) food is changed in the lab to resist pests and disease, increase its nutrients, or increase quality or shelf life. Forty genetically modified foods may be sold in the United States, including tomatoes and corn.

Scientists expect that genetic modifications will increasingly enhance the nutritional value of genetically modified foods. A genetically modified potato in the works contains lots of protein. Golden rice that contains DNA from a daffodil (which is rich in beta-carotene) could be used help combat the vitamin A deficiency that causes 250 to 500 million new cases of blindness each year, mostly among children living in Africa and Asia.

Genetically modified foods pose the same risks or benefits to human health as do other foods, including allergens, toxins, and compounds known as antinutrients, which inhibit the absorption of nutrients.

Before marketing a genetically modified food, company scientists seek to determine whether these foods pose any heightened risks. The FDA published guidelines in 1992 to ensure that companies worked with the agency to assess the safety of genetically modified foods.

The FDA, EPA, and USDA share oversight of genetically modified foods. Although current tests have been adequate for evaluating the few genetically modified foods that have, so far, undergone relatively simple compositional changes, new technologies are being developed to evaluate the increasingly complex compositional changes expected. No scientific evidence exists, nor is there even a hypothesis, suggesting that long-term harm, such as higher cancer rates or recurrence, results from these foods.

Food Additives

In its broadest sense, a food additive is any substance added to food. Legally, the term refers to "any substance the intended use of which results or may reasonably be expected to result—directly or indirectly—in its becoming a component or otherwise affecting the characteristics of any food." This definition includes any substance used in the production, processing, treatment, packaging, transportation, or storage of food.

Additives are used in foods for five main reasons:
- to enhance color (colorings or bleaches), or flavor (flavorings, flavor enhancers, or sweeteners)
- to improve consistency and texture (emulsifiers, stabilizers, and texturizers that keep foods creamy and mixed; thickeners; humectants that keep foods moist; leavening agents; and anticaking agents).
- to replace nutrients lost during food refining or milling
- to preserve and keep food from spoiling
- to provide leavening or control acidity/alkalinity

Facts about Functional Foods

Functional foods are foods modified (for example, fortified, bred, or bioengineered) to offer health benefits. The idea of vitamin-fortified foods isn't new, but scientists have taken the concept many steps further. Some examples of functional foods are already in supermarkets—calcium-fortified orange juice, herbal tea with antioxidants, eggs with vitamin E. Those creating functional foods hope that they can improve upon nature and develop foods that are even better for you than before.

Approximately 44 nutrients are essential for health, but thousands of phytochemicals may also provide health benefits. Researchers are growing a strain of broccoli with higher-than-normal levels of certain phytochemicals. More research is needed to determine whether fortified broccoli affects cancer development in humans.

Isoflavones are among the most exciting phytochemicals, according to some nutritionists. Found mainly in soybeans, they are credited with an array of health benefits, including lowering the risk of prostate, breast, and other major cancers. Bioengineers are isolating soy genes that create tumor-blocking chemicals and splicing them into wheat, corn, and other grains to create what they hope will be anticancer foods.

There are thousands of phytochemicals, and we don't know which ones are most effective for disease prevention. There isn't enough scientific evidence to recommend increasing your intake of a specific phytochemical to reduce your risk of cancer or any other disease. For example, we don't know if lycopene-enhanced tomatoes are going to make a difference in prostate cancer risk or if someone can ingest too much of the added substances.

More research is needed into functional foods. Meanwhile, eating a balanced diet that includes at least five servings of vegetables and fruits a day as well as grains and legumes will provide your body with a wide variety of phytochemicals.

Additives have been used for many years and have played an important role in reducing serious nutritional deficiencies among Americans. All additives are subject to ongoing safety review as scientific understanding and methods of testing continue to improve. (In fact, federal regulations for assuring safety of food additives are stronger than regulations that apply to dietary supplements.)

Food Additives and Common Uses

Additive Uses	Additive Examples	Foods Where They Might Be Found
To Improve Food Consistency	alginates, lecithin, mono- and diglycerides, methyl cellulose, carrageenan, glyceride, pectin, guar gum, sodium aluminosilicate	baked goods, cake mixes, salad dressings, ice cream, processed cheese, coconut, table salt
To Add Nutritional Value	vitamins A and D, thiamine, niacin, riboflavin, pyridoxine, folic acid, ascorbic acid, calcium carbonate, zinc oxide, iron	flour, bread, biscuits, breakfast cereals, pasta, margarine, milk, iodized salt, gelatin desserts
To Make More Palatable and Wholesome	propionic acid and its salts, ascorbic acid, butylated hydroxy anisole (BHA), butylated hydroxytoluene (BHT), benzoates, sodium nitrite, citric acid	bread, cheese, crackers, frozen and dried fruit, margarine, lard, potato chips, cake mixes, meat
To Improve Texture and Balance Acidity and Alkalinity	yeast, sodium bicarbonate, citric acid, fumaric acid, phosphoric acid, lactic acid, tartrates	cakes, cookies, quick breads, crackers, butter, chocolates, soft drinks
To Add Flavor or Color	cloves, ginger, fructose, aspartame, saccharin, FD&C red No. 40, monosodium glutamate, caramel, annatto, limonene, turmeric	spice cake, gingerbread, soft drinks, yogurt, soup, confections, baked goods, cheeses, jams, gum

Many substances that are added to food may seem foreign when listed on the ingredient label but are actually quite familiar. For example, ascorbic acid is another name for vitamin C; alphatocopherol is another name for vitamin E; and beta-carotene is a source of vitamin A. All food is made up of chemicals. Carbon, hydrogen, and other chemical elements provide the basic building blocks for everything in life.

Indirect food additives are those that become part of the food in trace amounts due to its packaging, storage, or other handling. (Food packaging manufacturers must prove to the FDA that all materials coming in contact with food are safe before they are permitted for use in such a manner.)

To market a new food or color additive, a manufacturer must first petition the FDA for its approval. Animal studies using large doses of the additive for long periods are often necessary to show that the substance would not cause harmful effects at expected levels of human consumption. Studies of the additive in humans also may be submitted to the FDA.

If an additive is approved, the FDA issues regulations that may include the types of foods in which it can be used, the maximum amounts to be used, and how it should be identified on food labels. Additives proposed for use in meat and poultry products also must receive specific authorization by the USDA. Federal officials then carefully monitor the extent of Americans' consumption of the new additive and results of any new research on its safety to assure its use continues to be within safe limits.

Additives are usually present in very small quantities in food, and no convincing evidence has shown that any additive at these levels causes human cancers or recurrence.

Irradiated Foods

Radiation is increasingly used to kill harmful organisms on foods in order to extend their "shelf life." Radiation does not remain in the foods after treatment, and consuming irradiated foods does not appear to increase cancer risk.

Many health experts agree that irradiation can be an effective way to help reduce food-borne hazards and ensure that harmful organisms are not in the foods we buy. During irradiation, foods are exposed briefly to a radiant energy source such as gamma rays or electron beams within a shielded facility. Irradiation is not a substitute for proper food manufacturing and handling procedures. But the process, especially when used to treat meat and poultry products, can kill harmful bacteria, greatly reducing potential hazards.

Irradiation does not make foods radioactive, just as an airport luggage scanner does not make luggage radioactive. Nor does it cause harmful chemical changes. The process may cause a small loss of nutrients but no more so than other processing methods, such as cooking, canning, or heat pasteurization. Federal rules require irradiated foods to be labeled to distinguish them from non-irradiated foods.

The FDA has approved irradiation of meat and poultry and allows its use for a variety of other foods, including fresh vegetables and fruits and spices. The agency determined that the process is safe and effective in decreasing or eliminating harmful bacteria. Irradiation also reduces spoilage, bacteria, insects and parasites. In certain vegetables and fruits it inhibits sprouting and delays ripening. For example, irradiated strawberries stay unspoiled up to three weeks, versus three to five days for untreated berries.

Food irradiation is allowed in nearly 40 countries and is endorsed by the World Health Organization, the American Medical Association, and many other organizations.

Organic Foods

The term organic is often used to refer to plant foods grown without pesticides and genetic modifications. It is also used to refer to meat, poultry, eggs, and dairy products raised without antibiotics or growth hormones. Organic food is produced without using most conventional pesticides; fertilizers made with synthetic ingredients or sewage sludge; bioengineering; or ionizing radiation.

The terms *natural* and *organic* are not interchangeable. Only food labeled organic has been certified as meeting USDA organic standards. The term natural has not been defined in FDA's law (the Federal Food, Drug, and Cosmetic Act) or in FDA's regulations.

The USDA has put in place a set of national standards that food labeled "organic" must meet, whether it is grown in the United States or imported from other countries. Before a product can be labeled organic, a government-approved certifier inspects the farm where the food is grown to make sure the farmer is following all the rules necessary to meet USDA organic standards. Companies that handle or process organic food before it gets to your local supermarket or restaurant must be certified too.

Organic food differs from conventionally produced food in the way it is grown, handled, and processed. Organic foods contain fewer contaminants than conventionally produced foods. However, the USDA makes no claims that organically produced food is safer or more nutritious than conventionally produced food.

Labeling Organics

What's in a label? Here are the differences when it comes to organic foods.

Foods labeled "100 percent organic" and "organic":

- Products labeled as "100 percent organic" must contain (excluding water and salt) only organically produced ingredients.
- Products labeled "organic" must have at least 95 percent organically produced ingredients (excluding water and salt). Any other ingredients must be nonagricultural substances approved on the National List or non-organically produced agricultural products that are not commercially available in organic form.
- Foods labeled "100 percent organic" and "organic" cannot be produced using excluded methods, sewage sludge, or ionizing radiation.

Processed products labeled "made with organic ingredients":

- Processed products that contain at least 70 percent organic ingredients can use the phrase "made with organic ingredients" and list up to three of the organic ingredients or food groups on the principal display panel. For example, soup made with at least 70 percent organic ingredients and only organic vegetables may be labeled either "soup made with organic peas, potatoes, and carrots," or "soup made with organic vegetables."
- The percentage of organic content and the certifying agent seal or mark may be used on the principal display panel. However, the USDA seal cannot be used anywhere on the package.
- Processed products labeled "made with organic ingredients" cannot be produced using excluded methods, sewage sludge, or ionizing radiation.

Processed products that contain less than 70 percent organic ingredients:

- These products cannot display the term "organic" anywhere on the principal display panel. They may identify the specific ingredients that are organically produced on the ingredients statement on the information panel.

A recent report indicates that organic produce may contain higher levels of antioxidants than traditionally grown foods. Anti-cancer substances seemed to be stimulated by the use of fertilizers. More research is needed to confirm these findings.

During cancer treatment some people may choose to eat organic foods when possible to reduce minimal exposure to pesticides. But keep in mind that further research is needed to determine whether organic foods are more nutritious or healthier for people with cancer compared to foods produced by other farming methods. Although many people are wary of synthetic chemicals sprayed on foods, 99 percent of the pesticides we eat occur naturally in plants.

Chapter 5

Dietary Supplements: Vitamins, Minerals, and Herbs

MANY PEOPLE WITH CANCER TAKE DIETARY SUPPLEMENTS such as vitamins, minerals, and herbs hoping to help halt or even reverse the course of their disease. Others take these supplements because of a desire to actively participate in treatment or a general desire to improve overall nutrition. In many cases, friends or family members encourage people with cancer to try the supplements. Some supplements, such as multivitamin/mineral capsules that meet United States Department of Agriculture (USDA) requirements, are useful and important. Other supplements may be touted as cancer treatments or cures. *No dietary supplement treats or cures cancer.*

Dietary Supplements

Dietary supplements are a diverse group of substances and products such as vitamins, minerals, and herbs that are not grouped together for any medical or scientific reason. Rather, Congress has lumped this diverse group of substances together based on the way it regulates these products.

According to the definition Congress established in 1994 in the Dietary Supplement Health and Education Act (DSHEA), a dietary supplement is:

> a product taken by mouth that contains a "dietary ingredient" intended to supplement the diet. The "dietary ingredients" in these products may include vitamins, minerals, herbs or other

botanicals, amino acids, and substances such as enzymes, organ tissues, glandulars, and metabolites. Dietary supplements can also be extracts or concentrates, and may be found in many forms such as tablets, capsules, softgels, gelcaps, liquids, or powders. They can also be in other forms, such as a bar, but if they are, information on their label must not represent the product as a conventional food or a sole item of a meal or diet. Whatever their form may be, DSHEA places dietary supplements in a special category under the general umbrella of "foods," not drugs, and requires that every supplement be labeled a dietary supplement.

In this chapter, we'll outline the risks and purported benefits of dietary supplements—especially selected vitamins, minerals, and herbs that people with cancer often read or hear about. As you read the rest of this chapter, there are two important things for you to remember:

1. While many dietary supplements may be touted as cancer cures, to date *there is no evidence that any dietary supplements are effective treatments for cancer.*
2. Particularly in the case of people undergoing treatment for cancer, *self-medication with dietary supplements can be risky and harmful.*

Risks of Dietary Supplements

Taking dietary supplements can be risky, especially for individuals receiving active anti-cancer therapy. Regardless of your treatment regimen, consult with your doctor and dietitian regarding the potential hazards and benefits of each supplement you are curious about—before ingesting even a single dose.

Doctors may not be familiar with the uses, risks, and potential benefits of some dietary supplements. Bridge this gap by gathering as much information as possible from reliable sources (see the rest of this chapter and the *Resources* section of this book for reliable information sources) on the dietary supplement therapy you are considering. Then approach your doctor with the information you have. Ask for his or her professional opinion as to whether the treatment is safe and medically sound, and how or if it might be safely integrated into your current treatment regimen. Take time to talk to other members of your health care team who are knowledgeable about supplements, such as dietitians. *Taking dietary supplements without consulting your health care team can be harmful and is discouraged.*

DIETARY SUPPLEMENTS CAN INTERFERE WITH CANCER TREATMENT AND PRESCRIPTION MEDICATION

Many people assume that dietary supplements can safely be taken along with prescription medication. Unfortunately, this is not always true.

Some supplements can change the way chemotherapy drugs or radiation treatment affects your body and can cause treatment to be less effective. For example, certain botanical supplements (supplements made from plants) can block or speed up the body's absorption of some prescription drugs, causing a person to have too much or too little of the drug in their bloodstream. Certain dietary supplements can cause skin sensitivity and severe reactions to radiation exposure. Patients undergoing chemotherapy are placed at significant risk for drug interaction if they take dietary supplements such as those containing high levels of antioxidants or folate. Some popular herbal supplements interfere with the blood's ability to clot (coagulate), and this effect is even stronger if you are on the prescription drug warfarin (Coumadin) or another blood thinner.

Most drug companies and producers of herbal supplements (supplements made from a plant or its leaf, root, or another part) do not conduct research on potential herb-drug interactions, so the risks of taking supplements with many medications are largely unknown. Herbs and drugs may interact and negatively affect your health or treatment. Talk with your doctor and dietitian about any herbal supplements you wish to take. They can tell you of any known interactions with prescription medications you may be taking and discuss the supplements with you. Discuss any changes in herb use with your doctor.

DIETARY SUPPLEMENTS ARE NOT STRICTLY REGULATED

All over-the-counter and prescription drugs are regulated in the United States by the Food and Drug Administration (FDA). However, because dietary supplements (including vitamins, minerals, and herbs) are *not* currently categorized as drugs, they are not subject to the same stringent safety and effectiveness requirements that pharmaceuticals are.

Manufacturers are not required to subject new ingredients or supplements to a series of clinical trials, which would demonstrate more clearly any risks and potential contraindications. Because Congress has decided to consider all dietary supplements "generally recognized as safe," they need not be tested under conditions that would put their risks and contraindications under the microscope.

The DSHEA gives the FDA permission to stop production of a dietary supplement, but only when the FDA proves that the product poses a significant risk to the health of Americans. The result is a system in which dietary supplements are assumed to be safe until they are proven unsafe. (Unlike supplements, the safety or efficacy of new drugs must be proven before they are available to consumers.)

Therefore, it falls to you, the consumer, to gather accurate information about the safe usage of dietary supplements, as well as about which manufacturers can be trusted to produce high-quality supplements. For more sources of information, see the information in the rest of this chapter and in the *Resources* section of this book.

THE GOVERNMENT CANNOT ENFORCE GOOD MANUFACTURING PROCESSES

The Department of Health and Human Services is in the process of developing a set of standards (called Good Manufacturing Processes or GMPs) by which dietary supplements must be manufactured. However, currently, there are no regulations or guidelines in effect for the production of dietary supplements.

The goal of the GMPs is to prevent the contamination and ensure high quality of dietary supplements. The GMPs for dietary supplements will be somewhere in between the tolerance standards for food production and the stringent consistency standards applied to drugs. Until these standards are put into effect, it is up to consumers to determine which products are safe and which are not.

The U.S. Pharmacopeia (USP) is an organization dedicated to producing quality control standards for the strength, quality, and purity of pharmaceuticals. In 1997, the USP began publishing standards for dietary supplements. These standards focus on the strength, quality, purity, packaging, and labeling of dietary supplements and are updated yearly. Manufacturers of dietary supplements are not required by law to adhere to USP standards. Supplements that are manufactured in compliance with USP standards are marked with the USP notation.

DIETARY SUPPLEMENTS CAN BE HARMFUL, ESPECIALLY WHEN SELF-PRESCRIBED

Like pharmaceutical drugs, dietary supplements have risks and side effects and can only be used safely within certain dosage guidelines. However, unlike drugs, dietary supplements are usually "self-prescribed" and administered with little or no input from informed medical sources. There is a lot of misinformation about the safe usage and potential risks of dietary supplements.

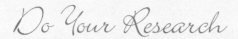
Do Your Research

When you're looking into using a supplement or researching any alternative treatment, keep in mind the following tips for finding reliable and helpful information about safety, interactions, and how to make your treatment as effective as possible:

- First, speak with your doctor or other health care provider about any supplement you are considering. He or she can probably tell you if the supplement poses any risks to your health and if the supplement is safe to take with other medications you may be taking.

- Be a skeptic. Most of what you hear or read about dietary supplements is based on anecdotal evidence—that is, evidence based on people's (even doctors') personal observations rather than on objective, controlled scientific studies. Much of the information you may encounter is produced by promoters and may contain biased or incorrect information. Be skeptical of sources that make grand claims based on a few people's testimonials or vague references to "scientific proof." Instead, rely on materials by trained experts on dietary supplements or the study of herbs (pharmacognosy). The rule "if it sounds too good to be true, it probably is" usually applies to such claims.

- Herbal and other botanical remedies have become an industry with billions of dollars in annual sales. The manufacturers of supplements have a vested interest in promoting their products. When researching your options, be aware of the manufacturer's hidden agenda: their bottom line.

- Find information on the product written by recognized medical experts or government agencies. Bring this information to your doctor's attention.

- If you are shopping for a botanical supplement, read the label carefully to determine which parts of the plant are used. Different plant parts contain different substances in different concentrations. Check information from reliable sources to see which parts are recommended. (Generally, health food store clerks are not recommended information sources.)

- Consider the name and reputation of the manufacturer or distributor. Is it a nationally known name? Large companies with a reputation to uphold are more likely to manufacture their products under strict, quality-controlled conditions.

- Rely on a trusted source such as the Memorial Sloan-Kettering Cancer Center's Herbs and Botanical Information web site (*http://www.mskcc.org/aboutherbs*) for reliable information about effectiveness, potential problems, and interactions. See the *Resources* section of this book for more sources of information.

Unfortunately, the misuse of dietary supplements or the use of dangerous supplements can lead to serious adverse reactions and even death.

The "Natural Is Safe" or "Natural Is Better" Myth

Despite the enormous progress in health care made possible by scientific understanding of how chemical substances interact with the body to treat various diseases, many people believe that a substance sold in its unrefined, naturally occurring state is better or safer than a manufactured or refined substance. However, supplements that claim to be "all-natural" are not necessarily better or safer for human consumption than refined or manufactured substances. Keep in mind that some of the most toxic substances in the world occur naturally. Poisonous mushrooms, for example, are completely natural but are not safe or beneficial to humans.

Traditional or historical use is, likewise, not a reliable gauge of safety. Tobacco was used for many years in Native American traditional medicine, but we now know it to be the cause of one third of cancer deaths in the United States. In considering traditional uses, it's important to pay attention to the details.

Most plants contain hundreds or thousands of chemical compounds, many of which influence functioning of the human body. Some of these compounds provide beneficial effects, while others can be toxic. Many drugs currently used in oncology and other fields of medicine come from plant sources. Based on decades of research, scientists have learned which plant components are responsible for the beneficial actions, and have separated these compounds from others that are harmful.

You should be able to get most if not all of the nutrients you need from food sources, especially vegetables and fruits. Physicians and dietitians may also recommend a single multivitamin/mineral supplement.

Some vitamin supplements may be described as "natural" or as "not synthetic." Scientists learned the chemical structure of vitamins decades ago. Most of these vitamins can be made synthetically (by chemical reactions of other substances). Whether a vitamin molecule is purified from a plant source or made in the lab, it has the same chemical properties and the same effects on your body. What is more important is that the product has consistent and accurate dosages, and that it is free of contaminants.

Claims: What They Mean and Don't Mean

Before you buy a dietary supplement, look at the label carefully. It is easy to mis-read the claims made about a product. The manufacturers of dietary supplements are allowed to make four kinds of claims on the labels of their products: nutritional claims, claims of well being, health claims, and structure or function claims.

Nutritional claims are statements about the effects dietary supplements, vitamins, and minerals have on known nutrient-deficiency diseases. For example, "vitamin C prevents scurvy." These claims do not need to be pre-approved by the FDA. However, the label must also make clear how prevalent the disease is in the United States to help consumers weigh the risk of contracting the disease against the potential risks of the supplement itself.

Claims of well being are just that: claims. Unevaluated statements about dietary supplements such as "makes you feel better" may or may not be factually accurate. Claims of well-being do not require pre-approval by the FDA or any other government agency.

Health claims are allowed to state the specific effects of a dietary factor on the body; for example, that "a diet low in sodium may reduce the risk of high blood pressure," that "oat bran and whole oat products reduce cholesterol," that "food containing sugar alcohol in place of sugar reduces the risk of tooth decay," or that "eating vegetables and fruits reduces a person's risk of cancer and heart disease." The FDA must pre-approve all health claims and requires that they be supported by evidence from scientific studies.

Structure or function claims are claims about the effect of the dietary supplement on the structure or function of the body that can imply but cannot specifically state their effects (for example, "beverages with antioxidants improve overall health," "grapes and grape juice support normal, healthy cardiovascular function," or "calcium builds strong bones"). The FDA published a ruling in January 2000 that clarified exactly what kinds of structure or function claims would be acceptable for dietary supplements. Dietary supplements may not make any claims regarding the treatment of disease. However, the following product descriptions are acceptable as structure or function claims for dietary supplements:

- the product's mechanism of action ("works as an antioxidant")
- the product's effects on cellular structure ("helps membrane stability")
- the product's effects on the body's physiology ("promotes normal urinary flow")

- the product's effects on chemical or laboratory parameters ("supports normal blood glucose")
- claims of maintenance ("helps maintain a healthy circulatory system")
- other non-disease claims ("helps you relax")
- claims for common conditions and symptoms related to life stages ("reduces irritability, bloating, and cramping associated with premenstrual syndrome")

Structure or function claims are the most controversial and the most confusing to consumers. They are not reviewed by the FDA and must be accompanied by the disclaimer: "*This statement has not been evaluated by the Food and Drug Administration. This product is not intended to diagnose, treat, cure, or prevent any disease.*"

The FDA requires this disclaimer on supplement labels because it is easy for consumers to misunderstand structure or function claims. For example, many consumers believe that a statement such as "helps maintain vision acuity" means the product has been proven to prevent vision deterioration or that one

Supplement Information: Rules of Thumb

- When you shop for supplements, look for the USP notation on the package label.
- Remember that a product described as "natural" is not necessarily safe or effective.
- Does the label provide a way to contact the company if you have questions or concerns about their product? (Many do not.) Reputable manufacturers will provide contact information on the label or packaging of their products.
- Try to avoid mixtures of many different supplements.
- Avoid supplements priced significantly lower than comparable products; they are likely to be of lower quality.
- Avoid products that claim to be "miracle cures," "breakthroughs," or "new discoveries," to have benefits but no side effects or to be based on a "secret ingredient" or method. Such claims are almost always fraudulent, and the product may contain potentially harmful substances or contaminants.
- Avoid products that claim to treat a wide variety of unrelated illnesses.
- Avoid dried teas and other dried medications sold loose in bags, often in street markets. They are often contaminated.

such as "helps maintain a healthy prostate gland" means the product has been proven to prevent or remove diseases such as prostate cancer. Be careful to avoid such misunderstanding; do not assume that because a product claims to support or promote healthy body function that it prevents or reduces the risk of any disease, including cancer. Recognize claims made by supplement manufacturers for what they are: untested, unproven, anecdotal reports.

Vitamin and Mineral Supplements

Vitamins and minerals are essential to health and are crucial in the normal functioning of our bodies. When you eat a balanced diet of vegetables, fruits, grains, dairy, and animal products, you get most of the vitamins and minerals you need in their most effective forms.

There's a world of difference between obtaining all of the vitamins and minerals you need by eating a balanced diet and taking vitamin and mineral *supplements*. Those who eat diets high in vegetables and fruits, which are rich in essential vitamins and minerals, have lower cancer risk, so it may seem that getting additional vitamins and minerals is more of a good thing. But there is no evidence that nutritional supplements can reproduce the benefits of a diet that contains vegetables and fruits.

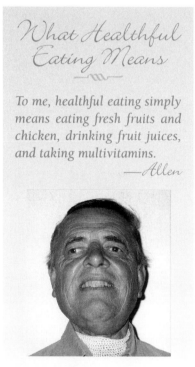

What Healthful Eating Means

To me, healthful eating simply means eating fresh fruits and chicken, drinking fruit juices, and taking multivitamins.

—Allen

Vitamins and minerals work together in the body in complex ways, affecting the absorption and processing of each other and in turn affecting the way the body runs. When you get vitamins and minerals through eating foods, the body is often able to maintain a balance of these nutrients.

Your dietitian, doctor, or nurse may advise you to supplement your diet with certain vitamins and minerals during treatment. This is especially true if you are unable to eat an adequate diet. In most cases, however, a multivitamin/mineral supplement that contains 100 percent of the daily requirements, along with calcium and vitamin D supplements, are sufficient and may be recommended by your oncologist. (For more information about dietary values like the RDA, DRI, AI, and DV, see the *RDAs, DRIs: Know the Lingo* section on page 10 of chapter 1.)

Misusing Vitamins and Minerals

Some people with cancer take large amounts of vitamins, minerals, and other dietary supplements in an effort to enhance their immune systems or even destroy cancer cells. There is no evidence to support this practice. Some of these substances can be harmful. In fact, as noted earlier in this chapter, large doses of some vitamins and minerals may reduce the effectiveness of cancer treatment.

The 1990s saw a trend of "megadosing" antioxidants such as vitamin C, beta-carotene, and vitamin E. Despite the fact that no scientific studies have ever proven that large doses of vitamin C can prevent or cure colds, many people still hold this belief. You may have heard a wide variety of claims about the benefits of taking large doses of certain vitamins. However, the practice of using large doses of vitamins to attack disease has no scientific basis.

Keep in mind the following tips when considering taking a multivitamin/mineral:

- Tell your health care team if you're taking a multivitamin/mineral or any other supplement.
- Expensive multivitamin/mineral supplements aren't necessarily better quality than generic or store brands.
- Make sure the label specifies that the multivitamin/mineral contains approximately 100 percent of the U.S. RDA of essential vitamins and minerals.
- Beware of ambitious claims for the multivitamin/mineral supplement's effects or any unusual ingredients.
- Talk to your oncologist to find out if you need any nutrients beyond a multivitamin/mineral.

If you are already taking supplements, bring the bottle(s) with you to your doctor for approval of the dose and to ensure that the ingredients do not interfere with your health or cancer treatment.

Antioxidant Supplements

Antioxidants are nutrients in vegetables and fruits that appear to protect cells in the body from free radicals. Antioxidants include vitamin C, vitamin E, selenium, carotenoids, and many other phytochemicals (chemicals from plants). Five or more servings of vegetables and fruits a day and a standard multivitamin/mineral supplement will give your body the nutrients it needs to stay strong and healthy. (See the *Phytochemical Power* section on page 26 of chapter 2 for more information about antioxidants.)

Taking large doses of antioxidant supplements may be dangerous and is not recommended while undergoing chemotherapy and radiation therapy. Several studies show evidence of potential interactions between antioxidant supplements (vitamins C, E, and A, for example) and radiation and chemotherapy. Since antioxidants protect cells from damage, or oxidation, they may keep cancer cells safe from oxidative cancer treatments, too.

Your health care team will develop a nutrition plan that meshes with your particular treatment regimen and will make decisions based on sound science. Talk with your health care team to determine the best time to take antioxidant supplements, and remember that large doses of any nutrient are not helpful and may be dangerous.

Limit doses of or avoid antioxidant nutrients only during cancer treatment. These beneficial nutrients can help both before and after therapy. But take them in moderation; where vitamins are concerned, more is not necessarily better.

Vitamins

Vitamins help the body use energy (calories) from carbohydrates, fats, and proteins. Bone strength, vision, and skin, nails, and hair are reliant on the vitamins you eat. Thirteen vitamins exist, each of which serves a different job in helping the body function.

Vitamins are either fat soluble or water soluble. Vitamins B and C are water soluble, which means our bodies can't store them and we need to take them in every day. Vitamins A, D, E and K are fat soluble, which means that the body can store these nutrients in its fat stores. (Fat-soluble vitamins can be toxic in large doses.)

Food and multivitamin/mineral packages list the Recommended Daily Amount (RDA) of each vitamin they provide. The RDA is what most people need to take in to stay healthy. People with cancer may have increased vitamin needs; your health care team can help you determine if you need more than a multivitamin/mineral to replenish your stores of vitamins.

Nutrient-Rich Snacks

Carrot sticks dipped in low-fat ranch dressing are not only tasty, they provide the beta-carotene you need.

—*Florence*

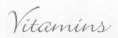
Vitamins

The primer below on vitamins shows food sources for the vitamins your body needs; what your body does with them when they're processed and put to use; supplement information; and some important scientific findings about supplements,

Vitamin	Natural Source
Vitamin A	It enters the body directly as vitamin A from animal sources, such as liver, fish-liver oils, and dairy products, and indirectly as beta-carotene—which the body converts to retinol—from many fruits and vegetables, including carrots, broccoli, spinach, squash, peaches, and apricots.
B Vitamins	*(see below)*
Vitamin B1 (Thiamine)	Vitamin B1 is found in cereals and whole grains as well as potatoes, pork, seafood, liver, and kidney beans.
Vitamin B2 (Riboflavin)	B2 is found in enriched bread, dairy products, liver, and green leafy vegetables.
Vitamin B3 (Niacin)	B3 is found in liver, fish, chicken, lean red meat, nuts, whole grains, and dried beans.
Vitamin B5 (Pantothenic Acid)	Vitamin B5 is found in almost all foods.

including studies, proven effects, and possible effects. Taking specific nutrient supplements during cancer treatment is not recommended unless directed by your doctor. Taking a daily multivitamin/mineral supplement that meets USDA requirements is a healthier idea than supplementing with various individual vitamins.

Function	Supplement Information
Vitamin A is essential for normal growth, bone development, reproduction, vision, the maintenance of healthy skin and mucous membranes (which line the digestive and respiratory systems, for example), and protection against infections in the respiratory, digestive, and urinary tracts.	High doses of vitamin A are toxic, and *long-term use of high dose supplements may increase the risk of lung cancer among people at high risk, such as smokers.* Large doses of vitamin A may increase the anti-coagulant (anti-clotting) effects of the blood thinner warfarin (Coumadin). Randomized clinical trials have indicated that *vitamin A supplements do not prevent recurrence or extend survival.*
B vitamins are essential nutrients for growth, development, and a variety of other bodily functions. They play a major role in the activities of enzymes (proteins) that regulate chemical reactions in the body.	*Current scientific evidence has not found any effect of B vitamin supplements on the growth and spread of cancer.* Overdoses can lead to heart and liver problems.
Vitamin B1 regulates enzymes that influence the functions of the muscles, nerves, and heart.	*Current scientific evidence has not found any effect of B vitamin supplements on the growth and spread of cancer.*
Vitamin B2 influences the production of energy in cells and health of the skin and mucous membranes of the digestive and respiratory systems.	*Current scientific evidence has not found any effect of B vitamin supplements on the growth and spread of cancer.*
Vitamin B3 also has a role in production of energy in cells and in maintaining health of the skin, nervous system, and the digestive system.	*Current scientific evidence has not found any effect of B vitamin supplements on the growth and spread of cancer.*
Vitamin B5 influences normal growth and development.	*Current scientific evidence has not found any effect of B vitamin supplements on the growth and spread of cancer.*

(continued)

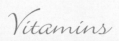
Vitamins

Vitamin	Natural Source
Vitamin B6 (Pyridoxine)	Fish, liver, pork, chicken, potatoes, wheat germ, bananas, and dried beans are good sources of vitamin B6.
Vitamin B7 (Biotin)	Vitamin B7 is manufactured by intestinal bacteria and is also present in peanuts, liver, egg yolks, bananas, mushrooms, watermelon, and grapefruit.
Folic Acid, Folate (Vitamin B9)	Green leafy vegetables, liver, citrus fruits, mushrooms, nuts, peas, dried beans, and wheat bread contain vitamin B9.
Vitamin B12 (Cobalamin)	Meats, fish, eggs, and dairy products contain vitamin B12.
Vitamin C (Ascorbic Acid)	Vitamin C is an essential vitamin that must be obtained from the diet, in citrus fruits like oranges, grapefruit, and lemons, and in green leafy vegetables, potatoes, strawberries, bell peppers, and cantaloupe.
Vitamin D	Only a few foods naturally contain significant amounts of vitamin D, including fatty fish and fish oils. In the United States, milk is fortified with vitamin D. Dairy products made from milk like cheese, yogurt, and ice cream are generally not fortified with vitamin D.

Function	Supplement Information
Vitamin B6 has an effect on protein, carbohydrate, and fat metabolism, and on maintaining health of red blood cells, skin, the nervous system, and digestive system.	*Current scientific evidence has not found any effect of B vitamin supplements on the growth and spread of cancer.*
Vitamin B7 helps break down protein, fatty acids, and carbohydrates.	*Current scientific evidence has not found any effect of B vitamin supplements on the growth and spread of cancer.*
Vitamin B9 influences growth, reproduction, blood-cell production, and the nervous system.	*Folate may protect against cancer, including breast, esophageal, prostate, bladder, and colon cancer. High doses of folate supplements can interfere with at least one chemotherapy drug, methotrexate.*
Vitamin B12 plays a role in growth, development, the production of blood cells, the functions of the nervous system, and how the body uses folic acid and carbohydrates.	*Current scientific evidence has not found any effect of B vitamin supplements on the growth and spread of cancer.*
Vitamin C helps bones and teeth form, helps resist infection, helps wounds heal, and is needed for blood clotting. Vitamin C is also an antioxidant, a compound that blocks the action of activated oxygen molecules, known as free radicals, which can damage cells.	*Vitamin C is selectively taken in by tumor cells. High doses (about 2,000 mg or more daily) may feed tumor cells, keeping them strong.* Do not take vitamin C supplements if you have kidney problems or if you are undergoing radiation therapy or chemotherapy (these therapies use free radicals to kill cancer cells, and vitamin C or other antioxidants may neutralize these free radicals and lessen their effect). *There is no evidence that vitamin C supplements provide benefits for people with cancer.*
Vitamin D maintains normal blood levels of calcium and phosphorus. It aids in the absorption of calcium, helping to form and maintain strong bones. It promotes bone mineralization.	There is emerging evidence that vitamin D may play a role in decreasing the proliferation of prostate cells. This may be due to its connection with calcium. High calcium intake may lower vitamin D levels, which may be the potential mechanism involved in prostate cancer. *The effect of vitamin D levels (or calcium levels) on people with cancer is not known.*

(continued)

Vitamins

Vitamin	Natural Source	Function
Vitamin E	The main sources of vitamin E in the diet are vegetable oils (especially safflower oil, sunflower oil, and cottonseed oil), green leafy vegetables, nuts, cereals, meats, egg yolks, wheat germ, and whole-wheat products.	Vitamin E is an essential nutrient that helps build normal cells and form red blood cells.
Vitamin K	Dietary sources of vitamin K, such as lettuce, kale, parsley, green tea, spinach, cabbage, broccoli, and turnip greens, as well as cereals, dairy products, some fruits, liver, and pork, provide the body with about half of the normal supply of the vitamin, while intestinal bacteria produce the rest.	Vitamin K is an essential nutrient the liver needs to form substances that promote blood clotting and prevent abnormal bleeding.

Minerals

Minerals stimulate the body's metabolic processes. The body needs only small amounts of some minerals, and eating a varied diet typically provides you with the minerals you need. The body stores nutrients for when you need them; this storage makes it possible to overdose on minerals in high-dose supplements.

Supplement Information

Supplements are not usually necessary unless the body has a deficiency of vitamin E, which can lead to a destruction of red blood cells and result in anemia. Excessive doses of vitamin E supplements taken over a long time can cause nausea, vomiting, stomach pain, and diarrhea. It has been reported that vitamin E at doses greater than 400 International Units (IU) per day may increase the effect of the blood thinner warfarin (Coumadin), although data are inconsistent.
There is no evidence that vitamin E significantly affects the growth of cancer

Only those who have symptoms of a vitamin K deficiency may need to take supplements. A deficiency may result from extended treatment with antibiotics (killing the bacteria that produce vitamin K) for several weeks or certain liver or intestinal disorders.
There is no evidence that a novel form of vitamin K is an active anticancer agent in human patients when used alone. More research is needed on a potent synthetic form of vitamin K and related compounds to determine if they may have any positive effects for people with cancer.

Cancer treatment like surgery and chemotherapy can diminish the body's stores of minerals. If you can't take in the minerals you need, your doctor may recommend a multivitamin/mineral or specific mineral supplement.

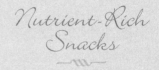

Nutrient-Rich Snacks

Almonds are some of the easiest nuts to digest, especially after sprouting for a day or two. They're an excellent source of protein, calcium, potassium, phosphorous, and magnesium They contain B vitamins and vitamin E. Sprouted almonds are crunchy and can be used in salads, dressings, bread loaves, cereals, and granola.

I like to soak a cup of almonds in water for a day, rinsing every few hours. Then I drain them and put them in a blender, adding soft tofu until it can be worked with a spoon. Then I spoon them into ice cube trays, freeze, pop out into freezer bags and save for smoothies, adding tofu, fruit, and soy milk.

—Joanne W.

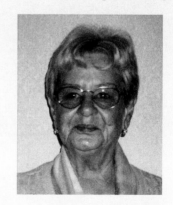

71

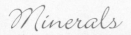

Minerals

The primer below shows some of the minerals that allow your body to function in many different ways. Some of these minerals show promise in slowing the growth of tumors. Others are often discussed by proponents as helpful for people with cancer, but no evidence of their effects has been proven. Use this chart as a guide to

Mineral	Natural Source	Function
Calcium	Calcium is found naturally in milk and other dairy products, leafy green vegetables such as broccoli and greens, nuts, seeds, beans, tofu (prepared with calcium), cheese, dried figs, kelp, oysters, and canned fish that still has bones, such as sardines and salmon. Because humans cannot make calcium, it must be obtained from diet or supplements.	Calcium is a mineral that is vital for a number of biological processes in the body, including heartbeat regulation. Calcium also contributes to healthy bones.
Copper	Copper is a trace element found naturally in foods such as seafood, organ meats, green vegetables, and nuts.	Copper assists in the regulation of blood pressure and heart rate, and the absorption of iron in the body.
Iron	Iron in meat, fish, and poultry is absorbed very efficiently by your body. Iron in plants such as lentils, beans, and flours, cereals, and grain products that are enriched or fortified with iron is not as well absorbed. (Consuming these plant sources of iron with sources of vitamin C can improve absorption.)	Iron is an essential mineral and an important component of proteins involved in oxygen transport and metabolism.
Magnesium	Magnesium is found in fish, whole grains, nuts, and leafy green vegetables.	Magnesium helps bones form and reduces the risk of osteoporisis, builds protein, and converts food to energy.

each mineral, where you can find it naturally in food, and the facts about each mineral's supplements. Again, taking mineral supplements is not recommended during cancer therapy.

Taking a daily multivitamin/mineral supplement that meet USDA recommendations is a safer idea than trying to supplement with various individual vitamins.

Supplement Information	Supplement Cautions
Calcium supplements will not slow the growth of most cancers, although they are being studied for the treatment or prevention of precancerous changes such as adenomas (polyps that may indicate future cancer growth) of the colon.	Calcium may interfere with the absorption of iron, fluoride, and zinc. Calcium supplements may increase the risk of hypercalcemia (an excess of calcium in the blood) for women on tamoxifen. *High consumption of calcium has been associated with an increased risk of prostate cancer.*
Human studies are needed to determine what role, if any, copper may play in the prevention or treatment of cancer.	Most people receive adequate copper intake from a normal balanced diet and do not require supplements. Copper toxicity is rare; however, a dosage over 35 mg/day is considered toxic.
Iron has not been tested for its effects on cancer or cancer treatment. A doctor may suggest iron supplements to alleviate fatigue for those undergoing chemotherapy.	Supplemental iron may cause gastrointestinal side effects such as nausea, vomiting, constipation, diarrhea, dark colored stools, and/or abdominal distress. Individuals with blood disorders who require frequent blood transfusions are also at risk of iron overload and should not take iron supplements.
There has been very little study of magnesium supplements and the body. *There is no evidence that magnesium supplements affect the incidence or development of cancer.*	People with kidney problems or blockage in the heart should not take magnesium supplements without a doctor's supervision.

(continued)

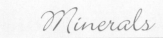

Mineral	Natural Source	Function
Molybdenum	Common sources of molybdenum include legumes, cereals, leafy vegetables, liver, and milk. Humans require very small amounts of molybdenum, which a well-balanced diet usually provides.	Molybdenum is involved in many important biological processes, possibly including development of the nervous system, waste processing in the kidneys, and energy production in cells.
Potassium	The body cannot manufacture potassium on its own and must obtain it from foods including apricots, potatoes, bananas, oranges, pineapples, green leafy vegetables, whole grains, beans, and lean meat.	Along with sodium calcium, and magnesium, potassium helps regulate major body functions, including normal heart rhythm, blood pressure, water balance in the body, pH balance (acidity and alkalinity), digestion, nerve impulses, and muscle contractions.
Selenium	The best nutritional sources of selenium are seafood, liver, kidney, whole grains, cereals, and Brazil nuts. Selenium is also present in drinking water in very low levels.	Researchers think selenium is an antioxidant, a compound that blocks the action of free radicals that can damage cells. Selenium may stimulate the formation of antibodies (proteins that help fight invading microorganisms) in response to vaccines. Selenium may also play a role in normal growth, development, and fertility.
Zinc	Zinc is found in lean meat, seafood, soybeans, nuts, pumpkin and sunflower seeds, eggs, cheese, and wheat bran.	Zinc (zinc gluconate, zinc sulfate) is a trace mineral that plays a key role in many bodily processes, including the building of DNA and RNA, energy production, cell metabolism, and regulation of the immune system.

Supplement Information	Supplement Cautions
Molybdenum deficiencies are very rare among humans; therefore most practitioners do not recommend supplements.	Some research indicates that high levels of the mineral can irritate the upper respiratory tract and cause swelling and deformities of the knees, hands, and feet. High levels may also cause gout.
Studies of the effects of a high-potassium diet on cancer have not shown a positive link between potassium intake and the prevention or development of cancer.	Excess potassium in the body can be toxic. Taking potassium supplements can cause potassium to build up in the blood, resulting in a condition known as hyperkalemia (symptoms include muscle numbness and tingling, abnormalities in heart rhythm, muscle paralysis, and possibly even heart failure).
Selenium shows promise as a nutrient that may prevent the development and progression of cancer; however, more research is needed. (See the *Selenium and Vitamin E* section on page 76 for information about selenium's potential effects on bladder cancer.)	Taking selenium supplements can be toxic to the human body if the supplements raise selenium levels beyond what the body can tolerate. No one knows for sure what that level is, however. High doses of selenium may also decrease the body's vitamin C absorption.
A few studies found that zinc levels in serum and/or inside white blood cells were frequently lower in people with head and neck cancer or childhood leukemia. Low zinc levels were also linked to increased size of head or neck tumors, more advanced stage of disease, and a greater number of unplanned hospitalizations. No randomized clinical trials have been done to show the effectiveness of zinc supplements in cancer prevention or treatment.	High doses of zinc can cause some serious side effects. An overdose of zinc can lead to a weakened immune system, vomiting, headache, and fatigue. *If you are taking fluoroquinolones:* Any zinc supplement should be taken either two hours before or four hours following the antibiotic drugs fluoroquinolones (for example, ciprofloxacin, levofloxacin, trovafloxacin, or gatifloxacin).

Selenium and Vitamin E: Bladder Cancer Enemies?

Studies have shown a link between high levels of selenium in the body and a lowered risk of lung, colon, and prostate cancer. One recent study shows that diets high in selenium can help prevent bladder cancer and are especially effective in preventing bladder cancer for former smokers. People in the study who took the highest levels of selenium cut their bladder cancer risk by approximately a third, and former smokers cut their risk of bladder cancer by up to 70 percent.

Vitamin E seems to have positive effects as well. A study of almost one million people in the United States reported that people who took vitamin E supplements over a long period had better survival rates when they developed bladder cancer than those who did not. Other lifestyle factors may affect this improved outcome.

Vitamin C didn't show a similar effect, which makes researchers wonder if vitamin E's antioxidant properties are involved, or another factor. A new study will examine the health effects of a combination of selenium and vitamin E in preventing prostate cancer. Observational epidemiologic studies have shown promising results. Meanwhile, the safest approach to getting your vitamins and minerals includes taking in healthful amounts of selenium and vitamin E from a balanced diet.

Herbal Supplements

There are two general groups of herbs: culinary herbs used in cooking to season food, and medicinal herbs used as remedies to treat illness. Culinary herbs are harmless when eaten in amounts typically used in cooking. Supplements contain much more of the herb than would be consumed through diet, and they can have powerful, often negative effects. The herbal supplements discussed in this book are very different from culinary herbs used to spice up meals.

Botanical medicine is the use of plants or plant parts in their natural state—without chemical processing—as medication for aches, pains, and illness. The herbs and other botanicals in these remedies contain many chemicals, and whether these remedies are helpful or potentially harmful often is not known.

Herbs are sold dried, finely chopped, powdered, and in capsule or liquid form. Products may include only the leaf, root, or another specific part, the entire plant, or a combination of different plants. They may be swallowed as tablets or capsules or brewed as teas. They may be marketed as single substances or in combination with other materials, such as vitamins, minerals, amino acids, and non-nutrient ingredients.

Herbs have been used to treat disease in every culture throughout the history of civilization. Today, herbs are found in a variety of products such as pills, liquid extracts, teas, and ointments. While many of these products are harmless and safe, others can cause severe and harmful side effects and interfere with proven cancer therapies including chemotherapy, radiation therapy, and recovery from surgery.

The herbal supplements we discuss are those most frequently asked about by people with cancer. They may be sold with claims of alleviating side effects of cancer treatment or as treatments for cancer itself. *Herbal supplements do not slow or reverse the spread of cancer. Herbs do not affect or control the growth of cancer or cancer cells.* People with cancer who are either in active treatment or who have completed therapy but who are considering herbal remedies, even for relief of symptoms or short-term problems, should first talk with their health care team.

Herbs should be avoided entirely during cancer treatment. They can interfere with chemotherapy and interfere with the blood's ability to coagulate during surgery.

Herbal Supplement Ingredients and Labeling

The basic difference between herbal supplements and medicines prescribed by a doctor is that herbals contain the entire plant or plant part, while prescription and over-the-counter medicines made by pharmaceutical companies contain only a purified active ingredient that has been studied and proven safe and effective. Many important prescription pharmaceuticals come from natural plants or herbs. For example, the following chemotherapy drugs are derived from plants: vincristine (Oncovin) and vinblastine (Velban) from periwinkle; paclitaxel (Taxol) and docetaxel (Taxotere) from yew trees; irinotecan (Camptosar) and topotecan (Hycamtin) from *Camptotheca acuminate* (a tree native to China and Tibet); and etoposide (VePesid) from mayapple.

(continued on page 80)

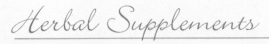

Herbal Supplements

Following is a list of herbal supplements that people with cancer may be curious about. Despite claims to the contrary, *no herbs affect or control the growth of cancer or cancer cells.*

Herb or Other Supplement	Claims
Asian Ginseng (*Panax ginseng*)	Claimed to prevent and fight diseases, including cancer; provide energy, and relieve anxiety.
Astragalus	Claimed to kill cancer cells, reduce chemotherapy side effects, enhance the immune system, and fight diseases.
Cat's Claw	Claimed to boost the immune system and be a remedy for cancer and other conditions.
Essiac	Claimed to strengthen the immune system, relieve pain, increase appetite, reduce tumor size, and extend survival.

Health Benefit or Harm	Scientific Findings
Possible hypertension, headaches, insomnia, restlessness; *estrogen-like effects could be dangerous for women with breast cancer history; do not use before surgery, with drugs that interfere with blood clotting, or with phenelzine sulfate, an antidepressant.*	*There is no scientific evidence that ginseng is effective in preventing or treating cancer.*
Abdominal bloating, loose stools, low blood pressure, and dehydration.	*There is no scientific evidence that astragalus can prevent or cure cancer in humans, decrease the toxic effects of chemotherapy, or enhance the effect of conventional immune therapy for some cancers.* Large-scale clinical trials are needed to test the potential immune-stimulating properties of this herb.
People taking certain medications, such as blood thinners, should not take cat's claw, nor should people who receive injections of foreign proteins (such as those taking medicine—for example, filgrastim (Neupogen)—to increase white blood cells or those being treated for anemia—for example, with epoetin alfa (Epogen).	No clinical trials have been conducted to evaluate the effect of cat's claw in humans. *No data exist showing that cat's claw is effective in preventing or treating cancer or any other disease.*
Do not take Essiac if you have kidney or liver problems or if you are in chemo-therapy (in one case, levels of a chemo-therapy drug were increased in the blood of a patient taking Essiac.) May have a laxative effect or cause increased urination; if taken with food, may cause headache, nausea, diarrhea, and vomiting.	No clinical trials have tested the health claims for Essiac. *There is no scientific evidence that Essiac is an effective treatment for cancer.*

(continued)

Herb or Other Supplement	Claims
Pau D'arco	Claimed to cure dozens of illnesses, including cancer, relieve infections, reduce inflammation, promote digestion, strengthen the immune system, and flush toxins from the body.
PC-SPES	Claimed to prevent or delay the recurrence of prostate cancer, inhibit the growth of prostate tumors, lengthen survival time, improve effectiveness of conventional treatments, and delay the need for chemotherapy.
Siberian Ginseng *(Eleutherococcus senticosus)*	Claimed to stimulate the immune system, increase energy, and quicken recovery from illness.

Because the FDA is not permitted to restrict distribution of a dietary supplement until there is already evidence that it has caused serious toxicities or death in humans, herbal remedy packaging is not required to provide information about its contents or possible dangers. Unlike approved medicines, herbs may contain harmful ingredients or contaminants along with those thought to be helpful. As

Health Benefit or Harm	Scientific Findings
Some of the ingredients are toxic; high doses may cause liver and kidney damage; low doses can cause vomiting and diarrhea and interfere with blood clotting. Do not take if you are taking blood thinning medication such as warfarin (Coumadin). *This herb should be avoided because of its side effects.*	*No well-designed, controlled studies have shown that this substance is effective against cancer in humans.*
Do not take PC-SPES if you are taking other herbal or dietary supplements (including grapefruit juice) or prescription medications. PC-SPES may increase their levels in the blood, which may result in toxicity. Do not take PC-SPES if you are on hormone therapy. PC-SPES may have estrogen-like effects and may alter your response to hormones.	PC-SPES lowers the levels of men's prostate-specific antigen (PSA), a protein made by prostate cells that is used to determine the presence and extent of prostate cancer. *More research is needed to determine whether PC-SPES is an effective and safe treatment for prostate cancer.* **RECALL:** PC-SPES was removed from the market by its manufacturer in February, 2002. The Food and Drug Administration (FDA) issued a warning to stop using this product. PC-SPES capsules were found to contain prescription drugs that could cause serious health problems. PC-SPES is not available at this time. New products made of many of the same herbs as PC-SPES are being promoted. Replacement products such as PC-PLUS have not been tested in clinical trials.
A few cases of diarrhea and insomnia have been reported; people with high blood pressure should avoid this herb.	*There is no evidence that demonstrates this herb's effectiveness against cancer.*

noted, many botanical remedies have not been scientifically tested, and there is little good or trustworthy information about their safety or effectiveness.

Check the product labels for both the quantity and concentration of active ingredients contained in each product. Consult the Memorial Sloan-Kettering Cancer Center's Herbs and Botanical Information site (*http://www.mskcc.org/aboutherbs*) to learn about acceptable ingredients and dosages.

Chapter 6

Diets Promoted as Cures for Cancer

A WELL-PLANNED DIET OF MAINLY PLANT FOODS and complex carbohydrates as a healthy basis for eating is supported by hundreds of scientific studies. Some diets may help improve your health by focusing on a combination of essential nutrients rather than too many fats and sugars, for example, but extreme dietary solutions don't cure cancer.

Diets Promoted as Cures for Cancer

Alternative or fad diets aren't supported by scientific evidence. Approaches that rely on enemas, fasting, or special supplements can be harmful, especially during cancer therapy, when getting enough nutrients is crucial. *There is no scientific evidence that any diet can cure cancer.* In this chapter we'll explore the evidence and assertions behind some of the most asked-about diets that may be promoted as cancer cures.

Abandoning conventional treatment in favor of any diet is likely to be detrimental to your health. Talk to your health care team about making changes in your diet and discuss how to make healthful changes a part of your care plan.

Regimens that Include a Special Diet

Some regimens promoted as cancer cures include diet as just one component of a treatment. Injections, medications, supplements, enemas, and other components may accompany a special diet aimed at curing cancer.

Livingston-Wheeler therapy is an unproven alternative cancer method that includes vaccines, antibiotics, vitamin and mineral supplements, digestive enzymes, enemas, and a vegetarian diet.

Livingston-Wheeler therapy is promoted primarily as a form of immunotherapy (a treatment that stimulates a person's immune system) that helps a person fight off serious illnesses like cancer. There is no evidence to support these claims.

Is there any evidence of benefit? *There is no scientific evidence that Livingston-Wheeler therapy is effective in treating cancer or any other disease.* This therapy has not been demonstrated to improve the quality of life for people with cancer. Few studies have evaluated Livingston-Wheeler therapy. One investigation involving seriously ill cancer patients found no difference in survival between patients receiving conventional treatment and those undergoing Livingston-Wheeler therapy. However, those patients receiving Livingston-Wheeler experienced poorer quality of life.

Are there any possible problems or complications? The safety of Livingston-Wheeler therapy has never been firmly established. Some reported reactions to the vaccine given in the therapy include aching, slight fever, and tenderness at the injection site. *Relying on this treatment alone and avoiding conventional medical care may have serious health consequences.*

Metabolic Therapies

Metabolic therapy involves using a combination of special diets and other elements in an attempt to remove "toxins" from the body and strengthen the body's defenses against disease. It is based on the theory that disease is caused by toxic substances that have accumulated in the body.

Metabolic therapists claim that metabolic therapy eliminates toxins and strengthens the body's resistance to invading microorganisms. Some practitioners claim that a special diet can cure serious illnesses, including cancer. Others claim that by evaluating a patient's metabolism they can diagnose cancer before symptoms appear, locate tumors, and assess a tumor's size and growth rate. There is no scientific evidence to support these claims.

Metabolic therapy varies a great deal depending on the practitioner, but all are based on special diets that usually emphasize fruits, vegetables, vitamins, and mineral supplements. Other components may include coffee enemas, enzyme supplements, visualization, and stress-reduction exercises, and Laetrile, a compound produced from almonds and apricot and peach pits. (There is no scientific evidence that Laetrile is effective in treating cancer or any other disease.)

GERSON THERAPY

Gerson therapy is a metabolic therapy. Practitioners of Gerson therapy believe that people with cancer have an excess amount of sodium that far outweighs the potassium in their bodies. Gerson therapy requires following a strict low-salt, low-fat, vegetarian diet, drinking juice from approximately 20 pounds of freshly crushed vegetables and fruits daily, and coffee enemas. Various other supplemental substances are injected or ingested to stimulate various organ functions, particularly the liver and thyroid.

Is there any evidence of benefit? *There is no scientific evidence that Gerson therapy effectively reduces cancer progression or improves survival, and it can be very harmful to the body.* There have been no well-controlled studies that support the beliefs and practices of Gerson therapy.

The National Cancer Institute and the New York County Medical Society reviewed the cases of several patients treated with Gerson therapy and determined that there was no evidence it is effective in treating cancer.

Are there any possible problems or complications? There are a number of significant problems that may develop from the use of this therapy. Serious illness and death have occurred from some of the components of the treatment, such as the coffee enemas that remove potassium from the body leading to electrolyte imbalances. Some metabolic diets, used in combination with enemas, cause dehydration. Serious infections from contaminated liver extracts may result. Thyroid supplements may cause severe bleeding in patients with liver metastases.

Participants in the Gerson program are required to discontinue conventional medical therapies. *Relying on this treatment alone and avoiding conventional medical care may have serious health consequences.*

Sticking to a Healthy, Balanced Diet

I investigated a number of options and decided that an overall healthy diet was one thing, but that some of the more focused and off-the-beaten path approaches were not right for me personally. I have always enjoyed eating and did not wish to make such dramatic changes in food and lifestyle without a guarantee of success.

—*Kathi*

Gonzalez and Kelley Treatments are metabolic therapies that use a combination of special diets and nutritional supplements in an attempt to remove "toxins" from the body and strengthen the body's defenses against disease.

Kelley's treatment includes up to 150 daily dietary supplements (e.g., enzymes and large doses of vitamins, minerals, and amino acids), fasting, exercising, and using laxatives or coffee enemas, a restricted diet, chiropractic adjustments, and prayer. Practitioners classify people into different metabolic types, which form the basis for specific dietary and supplement recommendations.

The Gonzalez treatment is similar to Kelley's treatment. Its focus is on detoxifying the body and bringing it into balance.

Is there any evidence of benefit? *There is no scientific evidence that metabolic therapy is effective in treating cancer or any other disease, or that the therapy is safe or effective.* Some aspects of metabolic therapy may be harmful.

There is general agreement that there are differences in the metabolism of cells in people with cancer compared to people without cancer. However, there is no evidence published in peer-reviewed medical journals that supports the claims made for metabolic therapy or any of its components. The treatment has not been shown to have any positive effects for patients with serious illnesses. Some aspects of metabolic therapy may, in fact, be harmful.

Several sets of researchers have reviewed the records of patients who used the Kelley therapy to determine if the therapy was beneficial. It was found to be ineffective, especially compared to conventional cancer treatment.

Dr. Gonzalez recently reported that in one (uncontrolled) study large doses of pancreatic enzymes increased survival times among patients with inoperable pancreatic cancer. This was a small pilot study conducted on ten patients. A randomized clinical trial sponsored by the National Cancer Institute is underway that is evaluating the use of pancreatic enzymes with nutritional support for treating pancreatic cancer.

Are there any possible problems or complications? Some aspects of metabolic therapy are considered dangerous. There are reports of complications related to liver cell injections and diets that contained too little salt. Several deaths have been directly linked to injecting live cells from animals (cell therapy). Also, a number of deaths have been linked to coffee enemas. Any diet containing raw meat or raw meat juice may be contaminated by bacteria. *Relying on this type of treatment alone and avoiding conventional medical care may have serious health consequences.*

Other Special Diets

Some treatments rely on certain foods and special methods of cooking—or not cooking food at all—to try to improve health. While a diet containing many vegetables and fruits, for instance, is often healthy, omitting animal products from the diet requires consuming other protein sources and getting a balance of nutrients such as B12, vitamin D, calcium, zinc, and iron.

VEGETARIANISM

Vegetarianism is the practice of eating a diet consisting mainly or entirely of food that comes from plant sources such as vegetables and fruits, legumes, and grains. Vegetarian diets vary widely. Some include no animal products (vegan), while others include dairy products (lactovegetarian) or dairy and eggs (lacto-ovo-vegetarian). Many vegetarianism proponents believe a vegetarian diet promotes health because it contains less fat, protein, and cholesterol and more fiber, vitamins, minerals, antioxidants, and phytochemicals than a diet containing meat.

All vegetarian diets include plant-based foods, such as grains, legumes, seeds, nuts, vegetables, and fruits, but vary according to the kinds of animal products consumed. One small group of vegetarians called fruitarians eat only raw fruits and fruit vegetables (like tomatoes) because they believe that cooking fruit damages its nutritional properties.

Currently, the American Cancer Society's (ACS) nutrition guidelines recommend a mostly plant-based diet that includes five or more servings a day of vegetables and fruits along with whole-grain products, nuts and seeds, and beans. The ACS recommends limiting your intake of red meats, especially those that are high in fat or processed, but notes that it is not necessary to avoid eating meat altogether after cancer.

Is there any evidence of benefit? Population studies have linked vegetarian diets with a decreased risk of heart disease, diabetes, high blood pressure, obesity, and colon cancer. Current evidence does not suggest that a vegetarian diet prevents cancer recurrence.

Many vegetarians are physically active and don't smoke, which may help improve their overall health and may account for potentially lower cancer rates. Eating a variety of vegetables is always appropriate, whether or not you choose a vegetarian diet.

Don't Count on Fasting or Juice

Juicing and fasting are sometimes combined into one therapy. Juicing therapy requires drinking the juice from vegetables and fruits rather than eating the vegetables and fruits themselves. Fasting involves not eating for a while, sometimes for a long time, although drinking liquids (such as water, tea, or juice) is permitted.

Fasting

Fasting is believed by some people to be an effective way of enabling the body to rid itself of toxins while promoting healing. Proponents of fasting for health rely on periods of not eating for several days to a month or more. By allowing the body to avoid the work of breaking down foods, those who fast hope the body will focus on healing and cleansing itself of toxins. Those who fast in hopes of treating cancer may hope to improve the immune system by reducing the work it needs to do and allowing it to fight cancer.

When people fast, water and fat are lost, but toxins actually remain. Fasting and avoiding taking in nutrients causes the immune system to suffer because it needs nutrients to run properly. Fasting also interferes with vital bodily functions and can damage vital organs. Rather than feeling sick because toxins are being released, as proponents claim, those who fast actually feel ill because not enough blood sugar is getting to the brain and other organs and they are unable to work properly. Fasting and causing blood sugar levels to drop also causes tissues to break down instead of producing energy—energy the body needs more of than ever during cancer treatment.

Are there any possible problems or complications? A totally vegetarian diet should be planned carefully to ensure that it provides all of the nutrients a person needs. If you eat a vegetarian diet during or after cancer treatment, be careful to guard against a nutrient deficiency. The more the variety of foods is restricted, the higher the risk is for deficiencies in important nutrients and for taking in too few calories for energy. Vegans, strict vegetarians who eat no animal products at all, must be careful to consume adequate amounts of protein, vitamin B12, zinc, and iron, as well as vitamin D and calcium. Getting ten percent or more of daily calories from protein (in foods such as dairy products—if they

Fasting can be a risky practice for people with cancer, especially for those malnourished by cancer. Researchers have found that the body cannot distinguish between fasting and starvation. Studies related to cancer suggest that fasting could actually lead to the promotion of tumors. *No evidence supports fasting as a healthy habit during cancer therapy or at any other time.*

Juicing

Juice therapies require that a person's primary sources of nourishment are fresh fruit and vegetable juices. Those who advocate juice therapy believe that this practice stimulates the immune system and helps the detoxification of the body.

The many health benefits of vegetables and fruits are well documented, but juice therapy is not specifically recommended. Juices are not sufficient as a sole food source, although they are great sources of nutrients when combined with a healthy diet.

Juices may be less filling than whole vegetables and fruits and may contain less fiber; also, fruit juice, in particular, can contribute lots of calories. Commercially juiced products should be 100 percent fruit or vegetable juices and should be pasteurized. Commercially prepared, unpasteurized juices and ciders may contain bacteria, which can be dangerous for people going through cancer treatment.

Juicing can add variety to the diet and can be a good way to consume vegetables and fruits, especially if chewing or swallowing are a problem or if your appetite is down. Juicing also improves the absorption of some of the nutrients in vegetables and fruits. However, juices alone won't improve the immune system.

are not vegan—nuts, dried beans, peas and lentils, and soy foods) is sufficient for most adults (elderly people may need more calories from protein, and people with kidney problems may need fewer). Regularly taking a multiple vitamin/ mineral supplement containing 100 percent of Daily Values or eating foods fortified with these micronutrients will help you get the nutrients you need.

Switching to a vegetarian diet may increase the amount of dietary fiber you consume, which could cause intestinal problems. Dietitians suggest a gradual rather than quick change in diet. *Relying on this treatment alone and avoiding conventional medical care may have serious health consequences.*

No Evidence: The Wheatgrass Diet

Wheatgrass is tall grass commonly found in temperate regions of Europe and the United States. The roots and rhizomes (underground stems) are used in herbal remedies.

Proponents claim that a dietary program based on wheatgrass commonly called "the wheatgrass diet" can cause cancer to go into regression and extend the life of people with cancer. They believe that the wheatgrass diet strengthens the immune system, kills harmful bacteria in the digestive system, and rids the body of toxins and waste matter.

There have been no scientific studies in humans to support any of the claims made for wheatgrass or wheatgrass diet programs.

MACROBIOTIC DIET

A macrobiotic diet is generally vegetarian and consists largely of whole grains, cereals, and cooked vegetables. Proponents of the macrobiotic diet claim that it can prevent and cure disease, including cancer, and enhance spiritual and physical well being.

Some vegetables are excluded. The diet also advises against eating fruits that do not grow locally, such as tropical fruits. Eating dairy products, eggs, coffee, sugar, stimulant and aromatic herbs, red meat, poultry, and processed foods is discouraged. Macrobiotic principles also prescribe specific ways of cooking food using pots, pans, and utensils made only from materials such as wood, glass, ceramic stainless steel, and enameled pieces. People who practice the diet do not usually cook with microwaves or electricity, nor do they consume vitamin or mineral supplements or heavily processed foods. In a macrobiotic diet, food is chewed until it is fluid in order to help with digestion.

Is there any evidence of benefit? *There is no scientific evidence that a macrobiotic diet is effective in treating cancer.*

Some research supports the health benefits of macrobiotic diets, but there have been limited studies of macrobiotic diet as related to cancer. The limited results available are controversial. No evidence indicates that following a macrobiotic diet reduces the incidence or recurrence of cancer more than following the ACS dietary and physical activity guidelines for cancer prevention.

Are there any possible problems or complications? Strict macrobiotic diets that include no animal products may result in nutritional deficiencies, such as an inadequate intake of protein, vitamin D, zinc, calcium, iron, and vitamin B12. The danger may be magnified for people with cancer, who often have increased nutritional and caloric requirements. *Relying on this type of treatment alone and avoiding conventional medical care may have serious health consequences.*

What we eat affects our bodies and our health and can even help prevent certain illnesses. But modern alternative therapies can be harmful if they require abandoning the nutrients your body needs, especially during cancer therapy when your immune system needs to be strengthened. Although the studies and testimonials shared by proponents of some modern alternative therapies may sound tempting and miraculous, purported dietary cures for cancer aren't based in scientific evidence. Follow the healthy eating guidelines recommended in this book to build and maintain a stronger, healthier body.

How Can My Diet Help Me Stay Strong During Treatment?

Chapter 7

Eating or Digestion Challenges during Treatment

URING YOUR TREATMENT, YOU'LL BE CONCENTRATING on fighting cancer. Eating well based on the nutrition information you've read so far will keep you strong and will supply your body with the nutrients it needs. In this chapter we'll discuss some ways you can prepare for treatment and for side effects.

Not everyone experiences side effects during cancer treatment. No one can predict how your cancer treatment will affect you, and until you begin treatment, you won't know exactly how you may feel. Many factors determine whether you will have side effects and how severe they will be, including the type of cancer you have, the part of your body being treated, the type and length of treatment, and the treatment dose. Your health care team can tell you more about your chances of having side effects and what you might expect.

Cope with Eating or Digestion Challenges

There aren't any hard and fast nutrition rules during cancer treatment. Some people with cancer may continue to enjoy eating and have a normal appetite throughout most of their cancer treatment. Others may have days when they don't feel like eating at all. For many people, side effects come and go. Adjusting your eating plan to stay well during treatment will help you handle your body's changing needs.

Eat a Healthful Diet

In this book, we use the terms "eating well" and "eating healthfully" to mean taking in a variety of foods that provide the nutrients you need while you're dealing with cancer. Eating healthfully provides you with distinct advantages:

- Eating a balanced diet allows you to enter and undergo treatment with reserves of the nutrients you need; these reserves help you keep up your strength, prevent body tissue from breaking down, rebuild tissue, and maintain your defenses against infection.

- People who eat well are better able to cope with side effects. You may even be able to handle higher doses of certain treatments than those who aren't eating healthfully. For example, we know that some cancer treatments are actually much more effective if the person with cancer is well-nourished and taking in enough calories and protein.

- Eating well is crucial in helping your body stay healthy. It's more important than ever that you eat healthfully as you undergo cancer treatment.

Treatment and changes in appetite and tastes may open some unexpected culinary doors; you may be surprised by some of the foods that appeal to you during treatment. Don't be afraid to try new things—you may never have liked certain foods before, but they may taste good to you during treatment.

Plan Ahead

Planning ahead will help you take advantage of time savers like food delivery, pre-planned menus, and friends' help with cooking or shopping. On days when you're feeling good, you may want to focus on eating meals with more nutrients so your body can store them for later use. If you have more energy than usual, consider cooking nutritious meals that can be divided into portions and frozen, then eaten on the days when you don't feel up to creating a meal from scratch. (For inspiration, consider the casseroles, soups, and other dishes in the *Recipe Resource Section* of this book.)

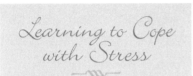

Learning to Cope with Stress

After being diagnosed and treated for prostate cancer, my stress level increased. Instead of losing my appetite, I sought out food during this stressful period. I had to learn to deal with my stress in more productive manners, rather than turning to food.

— Robert

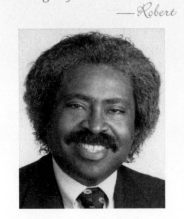

WHEN OTHERS COOK

Friends and loved ones may offer to pitch in with cooking duties—or may offer to get you out of the house for a meal on your feel-good days. Don't be stubborn or embarrassed to accept help. Others want to help and need to feel useful. Let them pitch in and help; it makes them feel good too. Some tips to make it easy for you to accept others' offers to help:

- Keep a stand-by grocery list on hand so it's easy to send a friend or loved one to the store or to order over the phone or Internet.
- Offer menus of foods that are to your liking for friends and family members who want to help.
- Keep a list of foods that appeal to you after treatment so those helping you will know what you can most easily tolerate.
- Take others up on offers to help prepare meals—and offers to clean up afterward.
- Eat out when you feel up to it. Feel free to ask about exact ingredients in a dish or the method used to prepare it.
- When you don't feel like going out, order from restaurants that deliver.

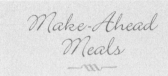

Make-Ahead Meals

When I feel well enough to cook I make many, many more portions than I can possibly eat at one sitting. I then divide the "leftovers" into tiny portions and freeze them. It's easier to eat healthily when I know something I like is already prepared and just needs to be reheated. (I do the same thing when someone brings me food.)

—Susan

GROCERY SHOPPING

Shopping during treatment can be difficult if you're tired, not feeling well, or if the smell of food doesn't appeal to you. Friends and family may be able to pick up and bring a few items to you as they do their own grocery shopping. If others aren't able to take over shopping duties, consider ordering groceries online if it's an option in your area or phoning in a grocery order to a store that delivers. When you do need to go to the store, get the most out of your trip by following these steps:

- Write out a grocery list in the rough order of the aisles you'll pass so you don't get sidetracked.
- Head to a small local grocery store so you can get through the store and lines more quickly.

- Visit a farmer's market if it is an option; you may cope better with food while shopping in the open air than you would in an enclosed store, where food odors are trapped.
- Buy multiples of items that won't go bad so you can reduce your trips to the store.
- Ask for help taking groceries to the car if you need it. If possible, shop when friends or family members will be available to bring in the groceries and put them away.

Ask your doctor, nurse, or a registered dietitian to help you plan meals and help you develop a grocery list of appropriate foods to rely on in case you have side effects such as constipation or nausea. (See chapter 12 for more information about coping with eating- and digestion-related side effects.)

STOCK THE REFRIGERATOR AND PANTRY

Ready your kitchen and pantry for your meal needs during treatment. Stock the pantry and freezer with many of your favorite foods so you won't need to shop as often. Include mild, easy-to-digest foods like gelatin, soup or broth, or hot cereal that you know you can eat even when you are sick.

- Purchase family-size or multiple individual portions in the freezer section of your grocery.
- Take advantage of prepared foods like washed and chopped salad ingredients, baby carrots, deli meals, boned fish and meat, and sliced cheese.
- Opt for some shelf foods that are easy to prepare, including couscous, canned soup, peanut butter, and tuna. These foods won't spoil and can help round out a meal at the last minute.
- Choose a variety of fresh, frozen, and canned fruits and vegetables. Many packaged vegetables are picked and canned or frozen right away, so they retain many of their nutrients.
- Keep the refrigerator, freezer, and pantry organized so that cooks not accustomed to your kitchen can find things easily.

In general, opt for meals with balanced amounts of meat, vegetable, carbo-hydrate, and dairy options so you can enter treatment with a healthful diet in place. Be aware that many prepared foods can contain a lot of salt and saturated or trans fats (fats in margarines, vegetable shortenings, and packaged breads, cakes, cookies, and crackers, similar to saturated fat in that they form artery-clogging deposits).

WHEN YOU COOK FOR YOURSELF OR OTHERS

After a cancer diagnosis, some home routines may need to change to accommodate appointments, treatment, and recovery. If you enjoy cooking for yourself or others, con-tinue doing so. Just be sure to make it easy on yourself by saving time and effort. Here are some ways to make cook-ing more pleasurable:

Simplify. Use kitchen appliances and gadgets to save time at the counter or stove. A food processor, slow cook-er, and microwave help you cook more efficiently and don't spread cooking smells throughout the house, in case you're feeling nauseous. Prepared foods, mixes, and frozen foods cut preparation time as well.

Stay flexible. When treatment begins, you may adjust your plan to make allowances for potential changes in taste or smell, a developed distaste for certain foods, or possible fatigue, for example. Keep in mind the nutritional advice in this book and offer a variety of nutrients in each meal.

Work together. If you cook and eat with friends or family, plan menus together so that everyone's tastes and nutritional needs are met. Share the grocery shopping, preparation, or cleanup duties—your friends and loved ones will likely be glad to help. Set priorities, especially if you're fatigued; concentrate on the planning or cooking if it's what you enjoy.

Label leftovers. Be aware of your refrigerator and freezer food supplies by noting the date and dish name on each container. (Cooked meats can be stored in the refrigerator—between 34 and 40 degrees F—for three to five days or in

Reduce Cooking Odors

I was fortunate to have a large freezer and caregivers who prepared meals for me that could be defrosted and cooked later. I discovered that on days when my nausea was at its worst, cooking with the microwave oven, rather than on the stove or oven in pots and pans, reduced cooking odors and controlled my nausea. Adequate cooking of foods is highly important, so I would caution that if you use the microwave, make sure that foods are fully cooked.

—Kathi

99

the freezer two to three months; raw meats can be refrigerated three to five days or frozen four to six months; cooked poultry can be refrigerated three to four days or frozen four months; raw poultry can be refrigerated one to two days or frozen nine months.)

Make meals enjoyable for you. Try to relax and enjoy your mealtime as a time to wind down, talk with others, or reflect. Use flavors you enjoy and add extra spices or seasonings to your portion if others don't enjoy the same tastes.

INVOLVE OTHERS

Talk to your friends or family members about helping with or taking over shopping and cooking while you're in treatment and may be fatigued or not feeling well. Others may also be glad to cook and freeze individual meals, cook double batches of the meals they prepare for themselves or their families, bring takeout from nearby restaurants, provide new recipes to try, and eat with you to make mealtimes more enjoyable.

You may want to consider having meals delivered to your home or eating a meal at a community or senior center. To learn more about meal delivery and other services, click on the "Contact Us" link at *http://www.cancer.org* or call 800-ACS-2345 for resources in your community. You might also look into support from county assistance groups, area churches, and social services.

Many personal chef businesses are cropping up around the nation. This service, which may include preparing meals on site or delivering premade meals, can be fairly expensive but can help you meet specific dietary requirements when your energy is low and nutrition needs are high.

Meals on Wheels Association of America is a membership association of programs that provide home-delivered and congregate meals. The goal of the organization is to improve the quality of life of those who need it. Some programs may provide other health and social services such as transportation, recreation, nutrition,

Create a Pleasant Atmosphere

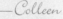

Put a flower or candle on the table, play your kind of music, and try to put your mind "out to lunch" while you eat. Eat with friends to distract you from any aversion to food.

—*Bertha (Birdie)*

Rely on Others

I have been very fortunate.... My partner (Kim) has been very supportive–she still goes with me to each appointment!

—*Colleen*

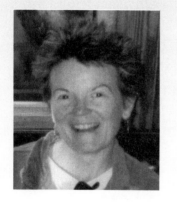

Time Saver: Cook and Freeze for Later

You may want to cook and store meal-sized portions of foods, especially before treatment times. After treatment you may not feel up to cooking. Keep in mind that:

- Many soups and casseroles freeze especially well, as do cooked lean chicken breasts, for example.
- Purchase small foil casserole containers that can go directly from freezer to oven.
- Undercook the meal you plan on freezing so it won't be overdone when you're ready to eat it.
- Freeze food as soon as it cools. Don't let it linger between 40 and 140 degrees F—the temperature range that allows bacteria to form.
- Label and date each meal and use it promptly, before it loses its flavor.
- Freeze washed fresh herbs and chopped, scalded onion for soups and casseroles. Wrap in a freezer-safe plastic bag for later use.

education, information, referrals, and case management. Contact Meals on Wheels at 703-548-5558 or *http://www.mowaa.org*.

Look Forward: Treatment and Eating-Related Side Effects

Many people have few or no side effects that keep them from eating. Even if you have side effects, they may be mild, and you may be able to control side effects with new available drugs—talk to your health care team about options that are appropriate for your situation. If you do have eating problems, you won't likely have them every day. And most eating-related side effects go away after cancer treatment is completed.

Treatment methods differ in their approaches to fighting cancer, and their side effects vary. Before treatment, it's a good idea to consider the potential effects of treatment on your body, your eating habits, and your digestion and to make a plan for coping with side effects if you encounter them. Although you may not need to implement them, planning ways to cope with possible side effects can make you feel more in control.

Conventional methods of cancer treatment—including surgery, radiation therapy, chemotherapy, hormonal therapy, and immunotherapy (biological therapy)—target the fast-growing cancer cells in your body. However, they can also damage healthy cells. The cells that normally grow and divide rapidly, such as those in the mouth, digestive tract, and hair, are often affected by cancer treatments. See the *How Cancer Treatments Can Affect Eating* section on the next page for some of the side effects that can occur as a result of cancer treatment. Later in this book, you'll read about specific side effects and what to expect, how to cope with them, and what to eat if you encounter them. For now, let's look at common side effects for each treatment and what to eat while you're undergoing treatment.

Don't be afraid to talk with the experts about your feelings and any concerns you have about treatment side effects. Your doctor and registered dietitian have helped many other people through successful treatment. When you understand your cancer and your treatment, you're less likely to encounter side-effect surprises along the way.

Surgery

Surgery, which removes cancer cells and surrounding tissue, is often combined with radiation therapy and chemotherapy to treat cancer. After surgery, the body needs extra calories and protein for healing and recovery. Many people have some pain and fatigue after surgery, and they may be unable to eat their everyday diet because of surgery-related side effects. (This can last for several weeks or months if the gastrointestinal tract is involved.) The body's ability to use nutrients may also be altered if any part of the mouth, esophagus, stomach, small intestine, colon, or rectum is surgically removed. Before surgery, discontinue any supplements that may affect the formation of red blood cells, thin the blood, or increase blood clots (such as vitamin B6, folic acid, vitamin B12, vitamin E, vitamin K, omega-3 fatty acids, garlic, and ginger).

NUTRITION SUGGESTIONS FOR PEOPLE UNDERGOING CANCER SURGERY

The day or night before surgery, you may not be allowed to eat or drink anything. After the operation, it may be several hours or even one or two days before you can eat normal foods and liquids. If you haven't eaten for more than a day or two, your doctor may advise you to start with easy-to-digest foods and beverages. (See the *What to Eat After Surgery* section on page 104 for more details.)

How Cancer Treatments Can Affect Eating

Cancer treatments can affect eating and digestion. Each person is different and not everyone has the same experience with side effects, but some side effects are most likely to affect you during cancer treatment.

Cancer Treatment	How it Can Affect Eating	What Sometimes Happens: Side Effects
Surgery	Increases the need for good nutrition. May slow digestion. May lessen the ability of the mouth, throat, and stomach to work properly. Adequate nutrition helps wound-healing and recovery.	Before surgery, a high-protein, high-calorie diet may be prescribed if you are underweight or weak. After surgery, some people may not be able to eat normally at first and may receive liquid nutrition supplements to help meet caloric needs or nutrients through a needle or a tube. Others may have mechanical limitations in the mouth, throat, or gastrointestinal tract as a result of the surgery.
Radiation Therapy	As it damages cancer cells, it also may affect healthy cells and healthy parts of the body.	Treatment of head, neck, chest, or breast may cause • dry mouth • sore mouth • sore throat • difficulty swallowing • change in taste of food • dental problems • increased phlegm Treatment of stomach or pelvis may cause • nausea and vomiting • diarrhea • cramps, bloating
Chemotherapy	As it destroys cancer cells, it also may affect the digestive system and the desire or ability to eat.	• nausea and vomiting • loss of appetite • diarrhea • constipation • sore mouth or throat • weight gain or loss • change in taste of food
Immunotherapy (Biological Therapy)	As it stimulates your immune system to fight cancer cells, it can affect the desire or ability to eat.	• nausea and vomiting • diarrhea • sore mouth • severe weight loss • dry mouth • change in taste of food • muscle aches, fatigue, fever
Hormonal Therapy	Some types can increase appetite and change how the body handles fluids.	• changes in appetite • fluid retention

Table courtesy of the National Cancer Institute, *Eating Hints for Cancer Patients*.

What to Eat after Surgery

An all-liquid diet may be prescribed just after surgery because it is easy to digest. If you have nausea, vomiting, or diarrhea, you may find it easier to get liquids into your system than solid food. A clear liquid diet is a short-term plan that includes only about 500 calories a day and doesn't supply adequate nutrients for long-term health. Once the gastrointestinal tract works normally and you resume eating enough to meet your nutritional needs, liquid nutrition supplements can augment the diet if inadequate nutrition is an issue. Meal "replacements" aren't a substitute for food; they improve or support nutrition when you can't eat enough calories or nutrients. Liquid nutrition can provide calories, protein, vitamins, and minerals.

Here is an example of a typical "diet progression" after surgery. If you have any questions about which step you should be focusing on, consult your doctor, nurse, or registered dietitian.

First Step: Clear Liquids

- plain gelatin
- weak tea
- strained citrus juices
- consommé
- strained lemonade
- clear, carbonated beverages
- juices
- bouillon
- popsicles
- water
- sport drinks
- clear, fat-free broth
- fruit ices
- strained vegetable broth

Second Step: Easy-to-Digest Foods (and all foods in Clear Liquids step)

- plain crackers
- white rice, noodles, potatoes
- all juices
- plain puddings
- plain milkshakes
- smooth ice cream
- carton or frozen yogurt
- white bread, rolls
- angel food cake
- soft or baked custard
- lean beef, fish, skinless chicken or turkey
- refined cereals
- milk, all types ice milk
- "instant" hot cereal
- fruit nectars
- canned, peeled fruits and vegetables
- strained, blenderized broth-based or cream soups
- pasteurized eggnog

Third Step: Regular Diet

- Be watchful of foods that cause gas: beans, melons, cruciferous vegetables, milk, and milk products.
- High-fat, greasy, or deep-fat-fried foods may not be well tolerated.
- Try to eat smaller, more frequent meals.

Some tips and suggestions for post-surgery eating and digestion:

- Foods and beverages that are low in fat and easy to digest are easier to tolerate than high-fat items such as fried or greasy foods.
- As you recover, make sure to take in plenty of fluids to prevent dehydration. Sip water, juices, and other clear liquids throughout the day.
- Eat as well as you can on the days when your appetite is good. It may be easier to eat small, frequent meals or snacks—start with aiming to eat half of a pre-surgery portion. Don't be too hard on yourself if side effects make it difficult to eat.
- Eat by the clock rather than waiting for hunger. Try to eat regular meals and snacks and try not to skip meals.
- Before treatment, you may have asked family and friends for help with shopping for groceries and preparing meals. Don't be shy about asking for regular help with schedules for grocery trips and cooking meals now.
- Try to resume your normal, day-to-day activities as soon as possible, with the guidance of your health care team. Ease into a more vigorous exercise routine carefully.
- Protein helps rebuild strength and create new cells. Include high-protein foods in your diet each day. (See the *How to Increase Protein* section on page 120 of chapter 8 for more information about protein-rich foods.)
- Make sure you get enough vitamin C, iron, calcium, magnesium, and potassium after surgery to aid in healing. (See chapter 5 for more information about foods rich in these vitamins and minerals.)

The type and duration of any side effects you have after surgery will depend on where in the body the surgery was performed and on your overall health. Drugs, self-care practices, and changes in diet can help lessen any side effects you may have. If side effects persist, be sure to alert your doctor, nurse, dietitian, or another member of your health care team and ask about ways to cope.

Radiation Therapy

In radiation therapy, radiation is directed at parts of the body with cancer so the cells are unable to grow and divide. While all cells exposed to radiation are affected by it, most normal cells can usually recover.

People with cancer usually receive radiation treatments five days a week for two to nine weeks. The type of side effects the therapy may cause depends on the area of the body receiving radiation, the size of area being treated, the total dose of radiation, and number of treatments. Radiation to the head and neck may cause redness and irritation in the mouth, a dry mouth, difficulty swallowing, changes in or loss of taste, nausea, and stiffness in the jaw. Radiation treatment to the chest may cause difficulty or soreness when swallowing. If you are having radiation treatment to the stomach or some part of the abdomen, you may have vomiting, nausea, or diarrhea. Radiation therapy to any part of the pelvis may cause one or more of the digestive problems listed above as well as heartburn, gas or bloating, or a low tolerance for milk products or other foods.

Side effects typically start around the second or third week of treatment and peak about two-thirds of the way through treatment. After radiation therapy ends, most side effects last two to three more weeks (but some may last longer).

If side effects develop, ask your doctor, nurse, or other health care professional whether medicines, a change in diet, or another change can help you manage them. (For more information about coping with specific side effects of treatment, see chapters 8–12.)

NUTRITION SUGGESTIONS FOR PEOPLE RECEIVING RADIATION THERAPY
Eating well while receiving radiation may be difficult if you are being treated at a facility far from your home. If you have a kitchen, you can store and easily prepare frozen foods, soups, or other meals.

If there is no kitchen where you are staying, keep foods on hand that do not need refrigeration, such as single servings of canned fruit, gelatin, puddings, cheese or peanut butter and crackers, granola bars, or cereal. In addition, remember to:

- Try to eat something at least 60 minutes before treatment rather than going to treatment with an empty stomach.
- Bring foods or commercial liquid nutrition supplements with you to eat or drink on the ride to and from treatment if you are traveling a long distance.
- Eat small frequent meals with fluids if food does not taste good, hurts going down, or causes diarrhea.
- Ask friends and family members to help with grocery shopping and meal preparation.

Do not expect to have the same side effects as someone else being treated for cancer in another area of the body. Even people undergoing the same type of treatment may have different side effects.

Manage Side Effects of Cancer Treatment

If you're having difficulty eating and have been following a special eating plan for diabetes or some other chronic health condition, talk to your doctor, nurse, or dietitian about how best to change your eating habits while you're having cancer treatments. To help manage side effects of treatment, consider the following tips:

- Try to eat small, frequent meals and snacks rather than three large meals. If your appetite is better at certain times of the day, plan on having your largest meal then.
- Nutrition supplements such as commercial drinks (for example, Carnation Instant Breakfast or Ensure) can be helpful during this time. Your doctor, nurse, or dietitian may have samples for you to try. Sometimes your insurance company will pay for nutrition supplements with a doctor's order.
- If you have thick saliva or a dry mouth, rinse your mouth often with a salt and soda mouthwash made of one teaspoon salt and one teaspoon baking soda added to a quart of water. Also rinse with it before meals and snacks.
- If you are having pain, diarrhea, or nausea, ask your doctor about medicines that will help.
- If you are having a great deal of difficulty eating, ask your health care team for tips to help you with eating.

Chemotherapy

Chemotherapy involves taking strong drugs designed to kill rapidly dividing cells. The drugs are most commonly taken by mouth or injected into the bloodstream. Chemotherapy drugs can damage both healthy cells and cancerous cells. Normal cells most likely to be injured are bone marrow, hair, and the lining of the gastrointestinal tract from the mouth to the rectum or anus.

Side effects will depend on what kind of chemotherapy drugs you take and how you take them. Common side effects of chemotherapy that can interfere with your ability to eat include loss of appetite, changes in taste and smell, mouth tenderness or sores, nausea, vomiting, changes in bowel habits, fatigue, low white blood cell counts (which increase the chance for infection), and changes in weight (gain or loss).

If you are having side effects from chemotherapy, tell your doctor or nurse. They may recommend medicines, daily self-care practices, and changes in diet to lessen eating-related side effects you are having. (For more information about coping with side effects, see chapters 8–12.)

Most people receive chemotherapy at an outpatient facility. A chemotherapy session may take anywhere from minutes to several hours.

You may be very tired while receiving chemotherapy. Fatigue (tiredness or lack of energy) is very common during chemotherapy. Vomiting can deplete the body's stores of vitamins and minerals. Ask your health care team about supplements or medications that can help alleviate fatigue. Unless you are given other instructions, eat a balanced diet that includes protein (meat, milk, and eggs) to help increase your energy. Other suggestions to reduce fatigue are to prioritize your activities, doing the most important when you have the most energy, and to balance rest and activity so that it does not interfere with nighttime sleep. For more information about coping with fatigue, see chapter 9.

Some tips that may make eating during chemotherapy easier for you:

- Plan ahead and bring a light meal or snack with you in an insulated bag or small cooler. Find out whether your facility has a refrigerator or microwave oven you can use.
- Make sure you eat something before receiving your treatment. Most people find that a light meal or snack before chemotherapy is well tolerated.
- Don't be too hard on yourself if side effects make it difficult to eat. Try eating small, frequent meals or snacks. Go easy on fried or greasy foods, which can be hard to digest. On days when you're feeling well and your appetite is good, try to eat regular meals and snacks.
- Don't be afraid to ask family and friends for help with grocery shopping and fixing meals.
- Try liquid nutrition supplements to add to the nutrients you're getting through food.

Some side effects of chemotherapy go away within hours of receiving treatment. If your side effects persist, tell your health care team. Prompt attention to nutrition-

Listen to Your Body

My wife Allyson was expecting our first child when I was receiving chemo treatment for cancer (we were often both nauseous at the same time). Unusual cravings for foods I had not eaten in more than a decade—like bolgna!—were a big surprise to me when no other foods seemed appealing. But I made that sandwich and it was the best thing I ever tasted!

—Tom

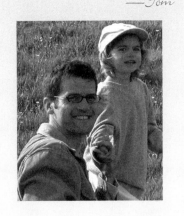

related side effects can help keep up your weight and energy level and help you feel better.

Immunotherapy

Immunotherapy, sometimes called biologic response modifiers or biologic therapy, is treatment to stimulate your own natural defenses of your immune system to fight cancer. Immunotherapy is sometimes used by itself, but it is most often used as an adjuvant (along with or after another type of therapy) to add to the anticancer effects of the main therapy.

Researchers have designed different types of immunotherapies to help the immune system recognize cancer cells and to strengthen the body's immune response so it will destroy cancer:

- Monoclonal antibodies are produced in large quantities in a laboratory rather than by the immune system. This type of therapy can be effective even if the immune system is weakened.
- Cancer vaccines contain cancer cells, parts of cells, or pure antigens (anything that causes the immune system to react, producing an immune response). The vaccine increases the immune response against cancer cells that are already present in the body.
- Nonspecific immunotherapies stimulate the immune system in a very general way. This overall increase in immune system activity can result in more activity against any cancer cells present.

NUTRITION SUGGESTIONS FOR PEOPLE RECEIVING IMMUNOTHERAPY
Potential side effects vary from treatment to treatment, but immunotherapy can cause fever, tiredness, and weakness, and can lead to loss of appetite and an increased need for protein and calories. If ignored, these symptoms can cause gradual or drastic weight loss (depending on the severity of the symptoms), which may lead to malnutrition (poor dietary intake). Malnutrition can complicate the expected healing and recovery process.

If you're experiencing a loss of appetite, eat high-calorie, high-protein foods when you do eat. Eating a nutritious diet including plenty of liquids may help fatigue. If you're coping with nausea and vomiting, don't force yourself to eat or drink, but try to sip water or clear liquids to prevent dehydration. Talk to your health care team about common side effects of your specific immunotherapy and how to meet your nutritional needs during treatment. (For more information about coping with specific side effects of treatment, see chapters 8–12.)

Nutritious Snacks

During cancer treatment your body often needs extra calories and protein to help you maintain your weight and recover and heal as quickly as possible. Nutritious snacks can help you meet those needs and help you maintain your strength and energy level and enhance your feeling of well-being. To make it easier to add snacks to your daily routine, consider the following if they fit into your dietary plan for treatment:

- Try to eat small, nutritious snacks throughout the day.
- Try to keep a variety of protein-rich snacks on hand that are easy to prepare and eat. These include yogurt, a bowl of hearty soup, cheese and crackers, peanut butter, egg salad, and tuna salad.
- Avoid snacks that may make any treatment-related side effects worse. If you suffer from diarrhea, for example, avoid popcorn and raw fruits and vegetables. If you have a sore throat, avoid dry, coarse snacks and acidic foods. (See chapter 12 for more information about coping with diarrhea and sore mouth or throat.)

Examples of Nutritious Snacks

• cheese	• nuts	• whole grain crackers
• peanut butter	• dips made with cheese,	• pretzels, popcorn
• eggnog (pasteurized)	beans, or yogurt	• puddings, custards
• fruit (fresh, canned, or dried)	• sandwiches	• egg salad
• soups (hearty)	• granola	• vegetables (raw, cooked,
• homemade milkshakes	• yogurt (refrigerated or frozen)	or juices)
and drinks	• ice cream	

Hormonal Therapy

Certain hormones (chemical substances released by glands that travel through the bloodstream and regulate body functions) influence the development and progress of some types of cancer, such as those of the breast and prostate. Hormonal therapy involves treatment with drugs that interfere with hormone production or hormone action, or the surgical removal of hormone-producing glands. Hormone therapy may kill cancer cells or slow their growth.

Some hormonal therapies can result in fluid retention, increased appetite, or weight gain. Other hormone treatments may cause mild nausea and fatigue. Talk to your health care team about side effects commonly experienced by people undergoing your specific therapy. (For more information about coping with specific side effects of treatment, see chapters 8–12.)

To cope with common side effects of hormonal therapy:

- Cut down on salt used in cooking and at the table to reduce water retention.
- Try to monitor your calorie intake to avoid excessive weight gain.
- Take medication as directed by your doctor to cope with side effects.
- Speak to your health care team to find out if calcium might help you retain bone mass and density during hormone therapy.
- Talk to your doctor and dietitian about taking products containing soy, phytoestrogens, and isoflavones to help alleviate hot flashes.
- Keep in mind that most of the side effects of hormone therapy are temporary and persist only during treatment.

Cancer, Healthful Eating, and the Family

Family caregivers are often eager to help the person with cancer feel better and regain his or her health. They may focus on the person's diet and weight—as well as the person's strength or physical activity—since they may be able to help manage these issues. A caregiver's sensitivity to the point of view of the person with cancer and a person with cancer's awareness of the caregiver's concerns may help prevent frustration on both sides about eating-related issues.

If people with cancer experience the side effects of treatment detailed in chapters 8–12 of this book, eating and keeping up their strength may be a challenge. Feeling ill or experiencing a decreased appetite may make people with cancer disinterested in food. Meanwhile their loved ones may be making efforts to provide nourishment and help them stay strong. Caregivers may think their loved ones aren't doing all they can to improve their condition,

Advice for Caregivers

Serve only as much food as the person with cancer has become accustomed to eating, not as much as you'd like for them to eat. Even if it's just a couple of spoonfuls, everyone will feel successful if the person eats all that is served—and there might be the reward of a second helping!

—*Kathi*

111

Keep Track of Side Effects

This form can help you keep track of eating-related side effects you may experience while you are undergoing cancer treatment. Feel free to copy this form and keep your own record. It may be helpful to share it with the doctor or nurse who is keeping track of your side effects.

YOUR NAME: _____ WEEK OF: _____

Measure your weight once a week: YOUR WEIGHT: _____ POUNDS

Write the type and date of your most recent treatment(s):

TYPE OF TREATMENT: _____ DATE: _____

TYPE OF TREATMENT: _____ DATE: _____

Keep track of eating-related side effects:

Some eating-related side effects people in cancer treatment may experience appear below. Check the box next to any side effect listed below that you experience in the week you have listed above. Next to each one you have checked, write a number from 1 to 3 indicating how severe you think each side effect was for you, where **1 = mild**; **2 = moderate**; and **3 = severe**.

Side Effect	Sunday	Monday	Tuesday	Wednesday	Thursday	Friday	Saturday
Sore/Dry mouth							
Nausea							
Vomiting							
Constipation							
Diarrhea							
Fatigue							
Decreased appetite							
Other: _____							

Other questions or concerns: (Use this space to write down questions or concerns you may want to talk about with your health care provider.) _____

_____

_____

fight to survive, or appreciate caregivers' efforts. People with cancer may feel a loss of control and may resent being treated as helpless or may feel that their caregivers aren't really listening to them. Keeping open communication and understanding common issues like this can help avoid such challenges and help both parties work to meet the needs the person with cancer.

Be careful not to make food issues the focus of the relationship between you and your family. Your loved ones may be concerned about your changed eating habits and may fear weight loss or other negative effects. Let them know that you appreciate their concern.

Cancer can cause role changes that require family members to be flexible and sensitive to each other's needs. If the head of the household or the person who traditionally took care of the grocery shopping, meal planning, and food preparation is ill, he or she may now be more dependent on other family members. Simple, healthful meals such as those in the *Recipe Resource Section* of this book are nutritious options during and after cancer treatment. Other tips for caring for the person with cancer are below.

COPING TIPS FOR CAREGIVERS RESPONSIBLE FOR FOOD PREPARATION
Anyone preparing food or meals for a person with cancer might want to remember these ways of coping:

- Be prepared for the person with cancer whose tastes change from day to day. Some days he or she won't want favorite foods because they don't taste good. Other times, he or she will be able to eat a dish that couldn't be tolerated just the day before.
- Have food within easy reach at home. For example:
  - a snack-pack of applesauce or pudding and a spoon on the bedside table if the person with cancer isn't feeling well that day
  - a bag of cut-up carrots in the refrigerator
- Have meals and snacks ready so the person with cancer can have something to eat when he or she is ready.
- Be prepared for times when the person with cancer is able to eat only one or two foods for a few days in a row, until side effects diminish. Even if he or she can't eat at all, encourage drinking plenty of fluids.
- Talk to the person with cancer about needs and concerns, and about ideas that might work best. A willingness to be flexible and supportive no matter what will help the patient feel in control of the situation.

❧ Try not to push the person with cancer into eating and drinking. Encourage and support without overwhelming him or her.

Chapter 8

"I want to maintain my body weight."

PEOPLE UNDERGOING TREATMENT FOR CANCER often gain or lose weight. It is becoming more widely accepted that being underweight or overweight may influence cancer outcomes. Therefore, paying attention to weight is very important for people with cancer.

Why Body Weight Is Important

It can be hard for people being treated for cancer and their health care professionals to tell the difference between healthy and unhealthy weight loss, and sudden weight gain or loss may indicate a health problem. Therefore all people in cancer treatment should aim to maintain their weight during therapy unless their health care team advises them otherwise.

Cancer and its treatments can cause gain or weight loss and may cause malnutrition. Many people with cancer lose their appetite at diagnosis, and many cancer treatments cause a loss of appetite as a side effect. For others, their treatment may limit the amount of or kinds of foods that they can eat. For more information about the high-calorie,

Eating to Prevent Weight Loss

During chemo, I loved potatoes every way, especially with cheese; rice with fresh broccoli and tomatoes; fruit drinks made of bananas, strawberries, and crushed ice; and lots of protein.

—*Becky*

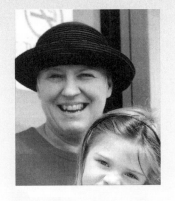

protein-heavy diet that is often recommended for people in cancer treatment, see page 13 of chapter 1.

When to Call the Doctor

Report weight changes of more than five pounds in a week or continuing weight loss of even one pound a week over more than two weeks to your doctor.

Remember that weight loss over time may affect your ability to function, leaving you weak and unable to participate in daily activities. In addition, unintentional weight loss or rapid weight loss usually reflects a loss of muscle rather than fat, which can place you at higher risk for malnutrition or depressed immune function and affect your ability to carry out normal daily activities. On the other hand, weight gain over time may result in a serious health condition, such as diabetes or high blood pressure.

While your weight does increase with fluid retention, this is not true weight gain. Be on the lookout for the following symptoms of fluid retention, and consult a doctor if you experience them:

- weight loss or gain of five pounds or more in one week or ongoing weight loss
- swollen ankles or feet
- shortness of breath
- dry skin or skin that "tents" when pinched
- excessive thirst
- dizziness

Weight Loss

You may lose weight as a result of cancer and its treatment. Weight loss can result from any of the following factors:

- the effect of the tumor, for example, growth in the abdomen and resulting discomfort
- psychological reasons such as depression and a resulting lack of appetite
- treatment—for example, surgery often causes weight loss for a few weeks, and biological therapy or immunotherapy may cause severe weight loss

🌿 treatment side effects such as nausea, changes in appetite, dehydration, or changes in how your body processes nutrients

Weight loss can cause fatigue, delay and lengthen recovery, suppress your immune system and make you more susceptible to infection, and negatively affect your quality of life.

COPE WITH WEIGHT LOSS

If you find that you are losing weight during treatment, try eating small, frequent meals and snacks every one to two hours. Keep handy high-protein, high-calorie snacks, and foods that are easy to take along when you are hungry. Also keep in mind these tips:

🌿 Some people going through cancer treatment may develop a distaste for fats. If this happens, try eating foods high in protein but low in fat, like yogurt, cottage cheese, eggs, and lean meat.

🌿 To increase calories but still get nutrients from fruits and vegetables when your appetite is down, concentrate your nutrients in dried fruits, 100 percent fruit or vegetable juice, or high-calorie produce like corn and peas.

🌿 Physical activity may help you reduce stress and increase appetite, but high levels of physical activity will make it harder for you to maintain or gain weight.

Consult your doctor if you experience any of the symptoms below that may accompany poor appetite:

🌿 nausea
🌿 inability to eat for a day or more
🌿 weight loss of five pounds or more
🌿 pain while eating
🌿 inability to urinate for an entire day
🌿 lack of bowel movement for two days or more
🌿 infrequent urination accompanied by pungent or very yellow urine
🌿 vomiting for more than 24 hours

How to Increase Calories

Cancer and its treatment often place extra demands on the body, causing you to need more calories than usual. Carbohydrates and fats supply the body with the bulk of the calories it needs. Here are some delicious ways to add calories to your daily diet.

Butter and Margarine
- Add to soups, mashed and baked potatoes, hot cereals, grits, rice, noodles, and cooked vegetables.
- Stir into cream soups, sauces, and gravies.
- Combine with herbs and seasonings and spread on cooked meats, hamburgers, and fish and egg dishes.
- Use melted butter or margarine as a dip for raw vegetables and seafood, such as shrimp, scallops, crab, and lobster.

Whipped Cream
- Use sweetened on hot chocolate, desserts, gelatin, puddings, fruits, pancakes, and waffles.
- Fold unsweetened into mashed potatoes or vegetable purees.

Milk and Cream
- Use in cream soups, sauces, egg dishes, batters, puddings, and custards.
- Put on cold cereal. Use in place of water in cooked cereals.
- Mix with noodles, pasta, rice, and mashed potatoes.
- Pour on chicken and fish while baking.
- Use as a binder in hamburgers, meatloaf, and croquettes.
- Use whole milk or half and half instead of low-fat milk.
- Use cream instead of milk in recipes.
- Make hot chocolate with cream and add marshmallows.

Cheese
- Melt on top of casseroles, potatoes, soups, noodles, and vegetables.
- Add cheese to meat, omelets, toast, and sandwiches.

Cream Cheese
- Spread on breads, muffins, fruit slices, and crackers.
- Add to vegetables or eggs.
- Roll into balls and coat with chopped nuts, wheat germ, or granola.

Sour Cream
- Add to cream soups, baked potatoes, macaroni and cheese, vegetables, sauces, salad dressings, stews, baked meat, and fish.
- Use as a topping for cakes, fruit, gelatin desserts, breads, and muffins.

- Use as a dip for fresh fruits and vegetables.
- For a good dessert, scoop it on fresh fruit, add brown sugar, and refrigerate until cold before eating.

Salad Dressings and Mayonnaise
- Use with sandwiches.
- Combine with meat, fish, and egg or vegetable salads.
- Use as a binder in croquettes.
- Use in sauces and gelatin dishes.

Granola
- Use in cookie, muffin, and bread batters.
- Sprinkle on vegetables, yogurt, ice cream, pudding, custard, and fruit.
- Layer with fruits and bake.
- Mix with dry fruits and nuts for a snack.
- Substitute for bread or rice in pudding recipes.
- Add to cereal, especially hot cereal.

Dried Fruits (raisins, prunes, apricots, dates, figs)
- Try cooking dried fruits; serve for breakfast or as a dessert or snack.
- Add to muffins, cookies, breads, cakes, rice and grain dishes, cereals, puddings, and stuffings.
- Bake in pies and turnovers.
- Combine with cooked vegetables, such as carrots, sweet potatoes, yams, and acorn and butternut squash.
- Combine with nuts or granola for snacks.

Eggs
- Add chopped, hard-cooked eggs to salads and dressings, vegetables, casseroles, and creamed meats.
- Make a rich custard with eggs, milk, and sugar.
- Add extra hard-cooked yolks to deviled-egg filling and sandwich spread.
- Beat eggs into mashed potatoes, vegetable purees, and sauces. (Be sure to keep cooking these dishes after adding the eggs because raw eggs may contain harmful bacteria.)
- Add extra eggs or egg whites to custards, puddings, quiches, scrambled eggs, omelets, and to pancake and French toast batter before cooking.

Food Preparation
- Add breading to meat and vegetables.
- If you aren't experiencing digestive issues, sauté and fry foods when possible, because these methods add more calories than do baking or broiling.
- Add sauces or gravies.

Courtesy of the National Cancer Institute, *Eating Hints for Cancer Patients*.

How to Increase Protein

Following treatment, your body usually needs additional protein to heal tissues and help prevent infection. Good sources of protein include lean meat, fish, poultry, dairy products, nuts, dried beans, peas and lentils, and soy foods. Here are some ways to add more protein to your daily diet to ensure that your body gets enough.

Hard or Semisoft Cheese
- Melt on sandwiches, bread, muffins, tortillas, hamburgers, hot dogs, other meats or fish, vegetables, eggs, desserts, stewed fruit, or pies.
- Grate and add to soups, sauces, casseroles, vegetable dishes, mashed potatoes, rice, noodles, or meatloaf.

Cottage Cheese/Ricotta Cheese
- Mix with or use to stuff fruits and vegetables.
- Add to casseroles, spaghetti, noodles, and egg dishes, such as omelets, scrambled eggs, and soufflés.
- Use in gelatin, pudding-type desserts, cheesecake, and pancake batter.
- Use to stuff crepes and pasta shells or manicotti.
- Add to salsa for a high-protein dip.

Milk
- Use milk instead of water in beverages and in cooking when possible.
- Use in preparing hot cereal, soups, cocoa, and pudding.
- Add cream sauces to vegetables and other dishes.

Nonfat Instant Dry Milk
- Add to regular milk and milk drinks, such as pasteurized eggnog and milkshakes.
- Use in casseroles, meatloaf, breads, muffins, sauces, cream soups, mashed potatoes, puddings and custards, and milk-based desserts.

Commercial Products
- Use "instant breakfast" powder in milk drinks and desserts.
- Mix with ice cream, milk, and fruit or flavorings for a high-protein milkshake.

Ice Cream, Yogurt, and Frozen Yogurt
- Add to carbonated beverages, such as ginger ale or cola.
- Add to milk drinks, such as milkshakes.
- Add to cereal, fruit, gelatin desserts, and pies; blend or whip with soft or cooked fruits.
- Sandwich ice cream or frozen yogurt between cake slices, cookies, or graham crackers.
- Make breakfast drinks with fruit and bananas.

Eggs

- Keep hard-cooked eggs in the refrigerator.
- Add chopped, hard-cooked eggs to salads and dressings, vegetables, casseroles, and creamed meats.
- Add extra eggs or egg whites to quiches and to pancake and French toast batter.
- Add extra egg whites to scrambled eggs and omelets.
- Make a rich custard with eggs, high-protein milk, and sugar.
- Add extra hard-cooked yolks to deviled-egg filling and sandwich spreads.
- Avoid raw eggs, which may contain harmful bacteria, because your treatment may make you susceptible to infection. Make sure all eggs you eat are well cooked or baked; avoid eggs that are undercooked. Alternatively, use refrigerated or frozen egg substitute made from egg whites.

Nuts, Seeds, and Wheat Germ

- Add to casseroles, breads, muffins, pancakes, cookies, waffles, and ice cream.
- Sprinkle on fruit, cereal, ice cream, yogurt, vegetables, salads, and toast as a crunchy topping; use in place of bread crumbs.
- Blend with parsley or spinach, herbs, and cream for a noodle, pasta, or vegetable sauce.
- Roll bananas in chopped nuts.

Peanut Butter/Seeds

- Spread peanut butter on sandwiches, toast, muffins, crackers, waffles, pancakes, and fruit slices.
- Use peanut butter as a dip for raw vegetables, such as carrots, cauliflower, and celery.
- Blend peanut butter with milk drinks and beverages.
- Swirl peanut butter through soft ice cream and yogurt.
- Sprinkle seeds on desserts such as fruit, ice cream, pudding, and custard.
- Serve seeds on vegetables, salads, and pasta.

Meat and Fish

- Add chopped, cooked meat or fish to vegetables, salads, casseroles, soups, sauces, and biscuit dough.
- Use in omelets, soufflés, quiches, sandwich fillings, and chicken and turkey stuffings.
- Wrap in pie crust or biscuit dough as turnovers.
- Add to stuffed baked potatoes.
- Mix diced and flaked meat with sour cream and spices to make dip.

Beans/Legumes

- Cook and use peas, legumes, beans, and tofu in soups or add to casseroles, pastas, and grain dishes that also contain cheese or meat.
- Mash cooked beans with cheese and milk.

Courtesy of the National Cancer Institute, *Eating Hints for Cancer Patients*.

Weight Gain

Some people, especially those with breast cancer, may gain weight during and after treatment. Weight gain is often unavoidable during treatment, and may result from treatment side effects (such as increased appetite and eating or water retention), treatment itself (such as chemotherapy, corticosteroids, tamoxifen, and other treatments and medications), less activity, eating in response to stress, treatment-induced menopause, or a combination of these factors.

Weight gain can contribute to fatigue, lowered self-esteem, depression, high blood pressure, and increased cholesterol. It may also increase risk of recurrence or another cancer. Weight management is very important for those with breast, colorectal, and prostate cancer.

COPE WITH WEIGHT GAIN

A healthful eating plan will meet your caloric needs but won't include many excess calories. (Look to the nutritional guidelines in chapter 1 for general rules of thumb on healthful eating.) Reduce your salt intake if your ankles are swollen. Increase physical activity as you are able to help maintain a stable weight. Even moderate physical activity (such as ten-minute walks around the block) can help improve your sense of well-being and strength and can keep your weight constant in times of stress.

Obesity is a risk factor for some of the most prevalent cancers in the U.S., including postmenopausal breast cancer and colorectal cancer. Both for this reason and because obesity is more and more common in the general population, many people are overweight or obese when they are diagnosed with cancer.

If you're interested in losing weight, talk to your health care team. They may want you to wait to pursue a healthful plan for weight loss until after you have recovered from treatment, or they may carefully monitor a modest weight loss program (with a goal of losing a maximum two pounds per week) and monitor any potential interference with treatment.

Maintain Body Weight by Cutting Fat

Substitute applesauce for cooking oil in baking recipes. Use fat-free yogurt instead of sour cream on baked potatoes and in mashed potatoes to cut down on your fat intake. (Note: This tip is appropriate for maintaining body weight when you are gaining weight during treatment, for example, for some women undergoing breast cancer treatment.)

—Ann

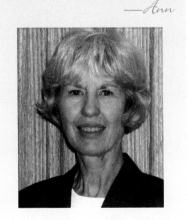

Nutritional Supplements

During treatment you may find it difficult to meet your nutrition needs through food alone. High-calorie and nutritional drinks can help pick up where your meals leave off.

Liquid nutritional supplements, which are often similar to milkshakes, come in many flavors. Some products offer a high-calorie option. (If the drink is too sweet, ask for one that is used for tube feedings, then sweeten the drink to your taste with syrups, blended fruits, or other taste enhancers. You may also want to try adding powdered coffee if you want to cut the sweetness of a drink.) Other nutritional drinks are similar to fruit drinks and can be mixed with ginger ale for variety. If you experience diarrhea, try the low-lactose and fruit-flavored nutritional drinks.

Another liquid nutrition option is Carnation Instant Breakfast, which is mixed with milk or mixed products to add calories and protein. Instant Breakfast doesn't provide as many nutrients as some other liquid nutritional supplements, but it is much less expensive. However, if you are sensitive to milk or know that you are lactose intolerant, you may want to mix with milk substitutes such as soy milk.

Nutritional products also come in bar and pudding form and can pack a nutrient punch.

Women treated for breast cancer who gain weight during treatment typically gain fat tissue but have either no change in or a decrease in their lean body mass. They may be able to effectively cope with this type of weight gain with exercise, especially physical activity that emphasizes resistance training or weight lifting.

Obesity has been associated with poorer prognosis of cancers of the breast and colon. There is also increasing evidence that being overweight increases risk for recurrence for cancers. If you want to lose weight during or after treatment, discuss your health and weight with your doctor and also with a dietitian, who can discuss your weight loss goals and evaluate your body fat percentage and your BMI (body mass index).

A safe weight loss plan for those in treatment or those who have completed treatment includes a healthful, well-balanced diet and physical activity tailored to your specific needs.

Ways to Cut Back on Calories

If you feel hungry between meals, drink water or low-calorie drinks or eat sugarless candy and fruit. Stock up on low-calorie foods for snacking and order healthful meals when you go out. (See chapter 13 for tips about controlling your portions and calorie intake when eating out after treatment.)

Smart Snacks at Home

Do not consume large volumes or too many portions of the snacks listed below. Even low-calorie items add up when eaten in large amounts:

- sticks of carrots and celery
- other bite-sized portions of vegetables
- sugarless gum
- low-fat cottage cheese
- apple slices
- raisins
- orange sections
- rice cakes
- sunflower seeds
- pretzels
- air-popped popcorn
- a variety of sugarless, low-calorie hard candies
- flavored decaffeinated coffee
- fruity or herbal teas
- lemon or lime water

Eat Out without Overdoing It

- Look for "heart-healthy" meals.
- Order a vegetable plate (avoid the casseroles and opt for "straight" steamed, baked, or boiled vegetables instead).
- Choose calorie-free beverages.
- Share one low-calorie appetizer and one entrée with a friend.
- Request sauces and dressings on the side so you can control how much you use.

Chapter 9

*"I want to have
more energy."*

F ATIGUE IS THE MOST COMMON SIDE EFFECT of cancer treatment. In fact, some estimates show that nine of ten people experience some fatigue during treatment.

Understanding Fatigue

Fatigue is different from the tiredness you might feel from the hustle and bustle of everyday life. This daily lack of energy can appear suddenly and can be overwhelming. It's not always relieved by rest. The following can be signs of fatigue:

- feeling like you have no energy
- sleeping more than usual
- not wanting to do normal activities
- not paying attention to your personal appearance
- feeling tired even after sleeping
- having difficulty concentrating
- lack of sexual desire
- feeling irritable or impatient

Most people don't experience fatigue once treatment ends, but some can feel fatigued for several months afterward. Treatment-related fatigue can affect many aspects of life, including your ability to take part in your usual daily activities.

Reasons for Fatigue

Fatigue during treatment can be related to the cancer itself or to side effects of treatment. Sometimes it's difficult to pinpoint the exact reason for fatigue. During treatment, cells are rapidly growing and dying. The many by-products created in this process make the body work harder to repair all of the damaged tissues and can add to fatigue. Consider the following treatment factors:

- Many chemotherapy drugs cause fatigue by destroying rapidly dividing cells like those in the bone marrow. This affects the red blood cells and can cause anemia, or a lower than normal red blood cell count. Fatigue is the most common symptom of anemia. If fatigue is due to anemia, fatigue can improve when the anemia is resolved through transfusions with red blood cells or by taking a medicine called epoetin alfa. This medicine is similar to a hormone in your body that helps the bone marrow produce more red blood cells.

- Radiation also destroys rapidly dividing cells and can cause anemia and fatigue, though anemia associated with radiation therapy is less common than with chemotherapy. Fatigue may last several weeks after treatment stops or may continue for several months.

- Biologic therapy can cause mental fatigue and ongoing physical fatigue.

- Some types of hormonal therapy may cause temporary fatigue.

Other factors related to treatment or side effects that may cause fatigue:

- Eating less and not getting adequate nutrition because of other treatment side effects (loss of appetite, nausea, vomiting, mouth sores, taste changes, diarrhea, or constipation, for example) can cause fatigue.

- Dehydration because of diarrhea or vomiting can lead to an imbalance in electrolytes (which are involved in the body's metabolism and help cells function normally), such as sodium, magnesium, and calcium, and can make you feel weak.

- Cancer cells may be competing with normal cells for nutrients, slowing the growth of normal cells and causing fatigue, along with weight loss and decreased appetite.

- Chronic pain can leave you feeling fatigued.

Keep Snacks Handy

Keep your energy up by eating enough. If you enjoy the computer, reading, or sitting outside watching the day go by, take food with you. Nibble on baby carrots while you type on the computer. Eat a few ham slices while you watch the birds at the feeder; eat chunks of apple as you read.

— Kathi

126

- Medications that help you cope with treatment side effects can also make you fatigued.
- Stress, feeling depressed, or not getting enough sleep during treatment can contribute to fatigue.

COPE WITH FATIGUE

It is important to figure out the cause of fatigue so your health care team can offer you appropriate treatment. Your health care team can help you determine what might be causing your fatigue and how you can best cope with it. Some ways you might alleviate or decrease your fatigue include adjusting your diet, reducing stress, and increasing physical activity. Other ways to cope with fatigue include:

- Plan rest periods to conserve energy for important things.
- Use light stretching and exercise to counter the effects of fatigue.
- Schedule necessary activities throughout the day rather than all at once.
- Get enough rest and sleep.
- Remember that fatigue due to anemia is temporary and that energy will slowly improve when blood counts return to normal.
- Let others help you with meals, housework, or errands.
- Don't force yourself to do more than you can manage.
- Gradually incorporate a daily routine of walking.

Call your doctor if you are unable to get out of bed for more than a 24-hour period, if you are confused, or if your fatigue is getting progressively worse.

Use Nutrition as Your Guide

Fatigue may be caused by poor nutrition and can be helped by eating with the goal of getting all the nutrients you need. You can eat for health by following general guidelines for nutrition and relying on a diet rich in plant-based foods. Eat to meet any increased nutritional needs you and your health care team have identified as well. Important parts of a nutrition plan to combat fatigue are sufficient calories and protein. (See the *How to Increase Calories* and *How to Increase Protein* tables in chapter 8 for specific foods you can count on.) Keep in mind the following important goals:

- Get enough calories. If your weight is stable during treatment, you need 15 calories for each pound you weigh. If you've lost weight, add another 500 calories to your daily intake. (If you weigh 160 pounds, you'll need 2,400 calories to maintain your weight; if you weigh 130 and have lost weight during treatment, you'll need 1,950 + 500, or 2,450 calories.)

The Keys: Calories and Protein

Taking in enough calories and protein may help alleviate or reduce fatigue. But how much is enough? Your dietitian can tell you your calorie and protein requirements and can set realistic goals. The actual amount of calories and protein needed by each person varies.

If you're doing light physical activity (for example, a quarter-mile walk, folding a load of laundry, planting a few flowers, making the bed, or cooking a light meal), the following formula can be used as a general guideline of how many calories are needed to maintain body weight while you're in treatment. If you're more active, you'll need more calories:

- underweight adults: multiply weight in pounds by 18
- healthy weight adults: multiply weight in pounds by 16
- overweight adults: multiply weight in pounds by 13

General guidelines for grams of protein needed by people with cancer:

- multiply weight in pounds by 0.5

Some people in treatment need more calories and protein. Your doctor, along with a dietitian who is familiar with the needs of people with cancer, can help determine your nutritional needs and options.

- ❧ Include protein. Protein helps heal and rebuild tissues. Protein from animal sources like milk and meat can help you get the amount you need. (Milk contains a gram of protein in each ounce of liquid; and meat, poultry, or fish contain 7 grams of protein in each ounce.) During treatment, a good rule of thumb is to get half a gram of protein for each pound you weigh. (If you weigh 160 pounds, aim for getting 80 grams of protein each day.)
- ❧ Get enough vitamins and minerals. Getting nutrients straight from food is ideal, since foods contain many other beneficial substances. But if you aren't taking in much food because of eating- or digestion-related treatment side effects, ask your doctor about taking a simple multivitamin that provides 100 percent of the recommended daily allowances of many nutrients. Always take multivitamins with food to prevent nausea.
- ❧ Stay hydrated. Drinking eight cups of liquid a day will help keep you hydrated. If you have side effects like vomiting or diarrhea, you'll need

When You're Too Fatigued to Cook or Eat Regularly

Eating nutritious foods, exercising, and resting may all be part of your plan to cope with fatigue. Learning to understand your patterns of fatigue and respect your body's limits may mean cutting back on commitments, adjusting your schedule, and really concentrating on taking care of yourself. Here are some ways to take advantage of your higher energy days and cope with low-energy days:

- Keep small portions of meals or leftovers so you can quickly heat and eat them.
- Eat your biggest meal when you're most energized and your appetite is greatest. If you're tired and not eating much in the evening, eat more at breakfast or lunch.
- Snack throughout the day to get in nutrients without having to face a big meal.
- Rather than skip a meal, drink a liquid nutritional supplement if you aren't hungry.
- Use prepackaged, chopped, and washed vegetables, precooked deli items, or frozen or canned foods to help with preparation time.
- Let family and friends help prepare food.
- Try eating after you've had a rest; your appetite may be greater then.
- Look into food delivery from restaurants or from Meals on Wheels.
- When you feel up to cooking, make a big batch of freezable food and save for later.

more liquids than normal. Water, fruit juices, milk, and broth count as good choices. Coffee and caffeinated beverages flush more water out of your body than other liquids, so steer away from caffeinated coffee, sodas, and teas.

- Talk to a dietitian. A dietitian can help identify which nutrients you're getting enough of and which you're lacking, and can help you create a balance in your diet that may alleviate fatigue. A dietitian can also help you cope with side effects that may be making it hard for you to eat and digest enough food to maintain a healthful weight. Nutritious drinks, which are available commercially, may help alleviate these side effects.
- Ask for help. If you're so exhausted that you can't eat, ask friends or family members for help. Ask your health care team about caregiver and other options that might help.

Other Ways to Cope

You can help conquer fatigue through non-dietary methods as well. The two ways of coping listed here, exercising and managing stress, complement each other as well.

PHYSICAL ACTIVITY MAY HELP

You may not feel like being very physically active during treatment, and you may be confined to bed because of cancer or treatment. Decreased activity can cause a lack of energy and a tired feeling.

Exercise slows down the release of stress-related hormones. Studies have shown that moderate physical activity on most if not all days can help you cope with anxiety and depression, improve your mood, boost your self-esteem, and lessen symptoms of fatigue as well as nausea, pain, and diarrhea. Even light physical activity can improve your appetite, aid digestion, and regulate bowel movements. Studies of women in treatment for breast cancer indicate that the many benefits of physical activity also apply for people in treatment for other cancers. There is good evidence that physical activity during treatment can help people cope with common side effects of treatment like fatigue, pain, or nausea, improve physical and functional well-being, and improve their overall quality of life. Keep in mind the following as you consider beginning an exercise program:

- Talk to your health care team about whether exercise is a possibility for you during treatment. Ask about any limitations or boundaries you should keep in mind.
- Don't overdo it. Start with activities that aren't too strenuous and set small goals, then build up to moderate exercise.
- Commit to exercising regularly, three to five times a week for 30 minutes—or with the frequency and duration your health care team recommends.
- Swimming, walking, and stationary bicycles are safer than other high-impact physical activities and may pose less of a risk of injury.

Regular Activity May Help You Cope

It was very helpful to maintain a normal routine of activities and a positive attitude. I worked out in the gym when I felt up to it (mainly brisk walking on a treadmill). Yoga and Tai Chi helped me deal with the discomfort of my treatments. I found that massage and foot reflexology were very helpful in making me feel more comfortable.

—Ling

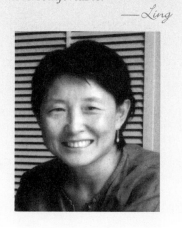

MANAGE STRESS AND DEPRESSION

Many people faced with cancer experience some degree of depression, anxiety, and fear. These are normal responses to a life-altering experience like cancer. You experience stress and worry if you aren't able to perform your usual family or work roles. You may be frustrated at not being able to "do enough." You may be upset from losing control over certain life events. You may be consumed by a fear of the unknown. When you're fatigued, such feelings can make you feel worse—and make you more tired.

Consider these options as you cope with stress or depression:

- Talk about your feelings and fears with loved ones.
- Remember that it is okay to feel sad or worried and frustrated.
- Seek help through counseling and support groups.
- Use prayer or other types of spiritual support.
- Consider physical activity as a method of coping.
- Take part in activities to distract you and keep you engaged.
- Try deep breathing and relaxation exercises several times a day. (Close eyes, breathe deeply, concentrate on each body part and relax it, starting with toes and working up to head; when relaxed try to think of a pleasant place such as a beach in the morning or a field on a spring day.)
- Talk with a doctor about using antianxiety or anti-depressant medications.

Don't keep your feelings inside or blame yourself for feeling worried or down. Your health care team can recommend someone who has experience helping people with cancer cope with their complex feelings. Feelings of sadness are normal when you have cancer. But sadness or emotional upset that lasts weeks or months or gets in the way of day-to-day functions may be clinical depression.

Depression doesn't always just go away, and it can be serious. If five or more of the following symptoms last for two weeks or longer, or are severe enough to interfere

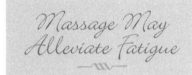

Massage May Alleviate Fatigue

Massage during my treatment helped me relax and provided me with some energy. I still love massage and would recommend it for anyone who is having chemo.

—Ivy

Have a massage one day before chemotherapy treatment. I found a massage therapist who really understood the special needs of chemo patients.

—Jan

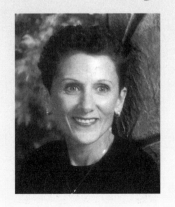

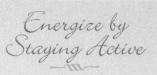

Energize by Staying Active

During my treatment period I accepted the offers of friends who wanted to visit me—it is very important to spend time with friends during treatment. I spent a great deal of time just enjoying what the city has to offer: going to movies, shopping, going to restaurants or just walking. Being out and about in the city helped to re-energize me.

—Ling

with your normal functioning, look into an evaluation for clinical depression by a qualified health or mental health professional:

- persistent sad or "empty" mood almost every day for most of the day
- loss of interest or pleasure in ordinary activities
- loss of appetite or overeating
- significant weight loss or gain
- inability to sleep, early waking, oversleeping
- restlessness or feeling "slowed down" almost daily
- fatigue, almost every day
- feelings of guilt, worthlessness, or helplessness
- difficulty concentrating, remembering, or making decisions
- thoughts of death or suicide, or attempts at suicide

Chapter 10

"I want to improve my immunity."

URING THE COURSE OF YOUR TREATMENT for cancer, there will be times when your body will not be able to protect you as well as it usually does. Some cancer therapies, such as chemotherapy and, rarely, radiation therapy, lower the number of white blood cells, which protect us against disease and foreign organisms. Cancer itself can also weaken the immune system. This immunosuppression (weakening of the immune system) means your body isn't as strong in the fight against infection and disease.

Your Immune System

The organs and cells that defend the body against infection or disease make up the immune system. Lymph nodes are bean-sized collections of immune system cells that are scattered throughout the body. Immune system cells are also found in the spleen (an organ found underneath the left ribcage), bone marrow (the soft inner part of bones where blood cells are produced), and in the digestive and respiratory systems. The immune system produces antibodies that recognize and kill some germs and mark other germs so various immune system cells and certain types of blood cells can destroy them. In other cases, germs are killed directly by the immune system cells working alone or together with blood cells. The major function of white blood cells is to defend the body against infections.

"Boosting" the Immune System

You may hear about supplements promoted to "boost" the immune system and help fight cancer. (The term "boost" may lead you to believe that a substance will increase the function of the immune system. But the word "boost" doesn't identify what a product does, and claims for "boosting the immune system" often aren't supported by evidence.) No such benefit has been proven. People with cancer—whether in active treatment or those who have completed therapy—considering taking any product that makes this claim should first talk with their health care team. For information about many of the substances below, see chapter 5. These herbals claim to "boost" the immune system:

- astragalus: There is no scientific evidence that astragalus can kill cancer cells or stave off illness.
- Echinacea: There is currently no reliable evidence proving Echinacea increases resistance to cancer or alleviates the immune suppression resulting from chemotherapy. (See the *National Institute of Health to Study Echinacea* section on page 146 of this chapter for more information.)
- cat's claw, Essiac tea, mistletoe, pau d'arco, and Siberian ginseng: all of these herbs are promoted as immune boosters that help fight cancer. No benefit has been proven.

Cancer Treatment's Effects on the Immune System

All cells need nutrients to grow and function. Dietary factors, such as decreased intake of vitamins, minerals, fat, calories, and protein, can alter immune function if cells do not have adequate nutrients to grow and perform this function. Poor nutrition makes the immune system less effective in recognizing and destroying germs, so people who are malnourished are more likely to develop infections.

People with cancer often don't get enough nutrients, and they may need more calories and protein to help their immune system cells and other tissues function properly.

SURGERY

Any type of major surgery can cause immunosuppression, but the reason for this is not totally clear. Within hours of surgery, researchers have noted decreases in immune function. Anesthetic agents may play a role in reducing immunity. Complete immune system recovery may take ten days to several months. Also, surgery often disrupts the skin and mucous membranes and exposes internal tissues to germs, thereby placing a person at an increased risk for infection.

Surgery is commonly used to diagnose, stage, and treat people with cancer. Factors that increase the risk of infection after surgery include the length of hospitalization, the extent of the surgery, the duration of the operation, the amount of bleeding during surgery, the nutritional state of the person, prior cancer treatment such as chemotherapy or radiation of the surgical area, and other medical problems a person may have, such as diabetes. People with cancer may be given antibiotics before surgery to decrease their risk of infection. The wound caused by surgery is a common site of infection. Because surgery is a common treatment for people with cancer, it is important to be aware of the chance of infection after surgery.

CHEMOTHERAPY

Chemotherapy is the most common cause of immunosuppression and myelosuppression (insufficient production of blood cells) in people receiving cancer treatment. The severity of immunosuppression and myelosuppression depends on the specific chemotherapy drugs used, the dosage, the schedule, previous treatments for cancer, age, nutritional status, type of cancer, and the stage of the cancer. Some drugs have a greater effect on the bone marrow (where red blood cells are produced) than others do. When chemotherapy drugs are said to be myelosuppressive, this usually means that the drug affects production of all blood cells. However, drugs may have different effects on the production of white blood cells, red blood cells, and platelets. Generally, white blood cell production is the most sensitive to chemotherapy drugs.

RADIATION THERAPY

The effects of radiation therapy on the cells of the bone marrow are similar to the effects of chemotherapy. Specifically, people may develop a low white blood cell count, which will increase their risk for infections. The total radiation dose, the radiation schedule, and the volume of productive blood cells directly in front of the radiation field (in other words, how much of the body is irradiated) affect the degree of leukopenia from radiation therapy. Unless people receive total body irradiation (TBI), they generally do not experience extremely low blood counts. This is because radiation is usually given to just one area of the body (chemotherapy, on the other hand, is systemic—it travels throughout the body). However, depending on the dose and type of radiation, the skin and mucous membranes may be damaged, making them less effective in keeping germs away from internal organs. Today, radiation treatments are given over many scheduled sessions rather than in one large dose. This has helped to decrease the amount of immunosuppression and risk of infections.

IMMUNOTHERAPY

Immunotherapy or biologic therapy is intended to improve the immune system's ability to recognize and attack cancer cells. Although these treatments stimulate immune reactions against cancer cells, they sometimes interfere with immunity against infections. People who receive immunotherapy may be at risk for immunosuppression and a low white blood cell count.

Food Safety

When your immune system is weak, the first step in staying free from infection is being aware of the bacteria and other organisms that could make you ill and steering clear or getting rid of them. The choices you make when buying and handling foods, preparing meals, and dining out can affect your susceptibility to infections. Following food safety guidelines reduces your risk of infection.

FOOD SAFETY AT HOME

Look at the lists here and keep in mind these simple ways of staying healthy when your immune system is weak. For example, avoid yogurt and ice cream products dispensed from soft-serve machines. Eat only well-cooked foods, avoiding raw and undercooked foods. And use defrosted foods right away without refreezing them.

The nutrition and food safety suggestions on pages 136–143 of this chapter (from A Guide to Good Nutrition During Cancer Treatment, Fourth Edition by Saundra Aker and Polly Lenssen and patient materials developed by Fred Hutchinson Cancer Research Center and the Seattle Cancer Care Alliance in Seattle, Washington; copyrighted materials) were developed for general oncology and bone marrow transplant patients who have weak immune systems. You may want to follow them, with your doctor's approval, while you are undergoing chemotherapy.

- Personal hygiene:
  - Wash hands frequently—before and after each step of food preparation— with plenty of soap and hot, running water for at least 20 seconds.
  - Wash hands before eating and after using the restroom, handling garbage, or touching pets.

🐾 Preparing foods:
- Use different knives to cut meat, produce, and bread.
- Do not taste food with the same utensil used for stirring.
- Wash fruits and vegetables thoroughly under clean, cold running water just before use (do not use produce rinses, soaps, detergents, or chlorine bleach solutions; produce may absorb these cleaning agents).
- Individually rinse the leaves of leafy vegetables such as lettuce or cabbage. Wash all packaged salads and other prepared produce under clean, cold running water, even when marked as prewashed. (Check the "use by" dates on packaged and prepared produce.)
- Wash the outside of all fruits and vegetables (such as oranges, melons, and bananas), even if the produce will be peeled or cut. This will prevent any bacteria on the outside of the fruit from being transferred to the fruit itself.
- Wash the tops of canned foods before opening, and clean the can opener after each use.

🐾 Thawing and cooking foods:
- Cook eggs until yolk and white are firm; cook egg dishes, custards, egg sauces, and casseroles that include eggs to a minimum internal temperature of 160 degrees F.
- Cook meats until no longer pink and the juices run clear. The only way you can be sure that meat has been cooked to a safe temperature is by using a food thermometer and the *Recommended Minimum Cooking Temperatures* on page 138 as guides.
- Heat leftovers to 165 degrees F.
- Thaw meat, fish, or poultry in the refrigerator away from raw fruits and vegetables and other prepared foods. Place on a dish to catch drips. Cook defrosted meat right away; do not refreeze. If you are in a hurry, you may thaw meat in the microwave, but cook it immediately after thawing.
- When microwaving, rotate the dish a quarter turn once or twice during cooking if there is no turntable in the microwave oven. This prevents "cold spots" in food where bacteria can survive.
- Use a lid or vented plastic wrap to thoroughly heat leftovers in the microwave. Stir several times during reheating. When food is heated thoroughly (to a minimum of 165 degrees F), cover and let sit two minutes before serving.

Recommended Minimum Cooking Temperatures for Egg, Meats, Poultry, and Seafood

	Product	Cooking Temperature
Eggs, Egg Dishes, and Casseroles	Eggs	Cook until yolk and white are firm
	Casseroles, egg dishes, custard, egg sauces	160 degrees F
Veal, Beef, Pork, Lamb, Rabbit, Goat, Game	Whole pieces of meat, hot dogs	160 degrees F
	Ground veal, beef, lamb, pork, rabbit, goat, game	160 degrees F
Poultry (Chicken, Turkey, Duck, Goose)	Chicken and turkey: whole bird and dark meat (thigh, wing)	180 degrees F
	Breast, roast	170 degrees F
	Ground chicken, turkey	165 degrees F
	Stuffing (always cook in separate container outside of bird)	165 degrees F
Ham	Fresh (raw)	160 degrees F
	Pre-cooked (to reheat)	160 degrees F
Seafood	Fin fish (such as salmon, cod, halibut, snapper, sole, bass, trout	Cook until opaque and flakes easily with a fork
	Shrimp, lobster, crab	Should turn red and flesh should become pearly opaque
	Scallops	Should turn milk white or opaque and firm
	Clams, mussels, oysters	Cook until shells open (may be high risk food for people with low white blood cell count or immunosuppressed)
"Ready-to-Eat" Meats	Hot dogs, luncheon meats, cold cuts, "deli-style" meats	Heat thoroughly until steaming

From *A Guide to Good Nutrition During Cancer Treatment*, Fourth Edition by Saundra Aker and Polly Lenssen and patient materials developed by Fred Hutchinson Cancer Research Center and the Seattle Cancer Care Alliance.

- Boil tofu, in half-inch cubes, for five minutes before using. (This process is not necessary if using commercial tofu in shelf-stable packaging—refrigeration is not needed until the product is opened.)

- Refrigerating and storing foods:
  - Purchase and use a food and refrigerator thermometer (available at many grocery and hardware stores). Hold foods at safe temperatures: cold food below 40 degrees F and hot foods above 140 degrees F.
  - Never leave perishable food out of the refrigerator for over two hours; throw away food left out longer than two hours.
  - Refrigerate fruits and vegetables. Discard fruits and vegetables that are slimy or show mold.
  - *Throw out foods that look or smell strange. Never taste them!*

- Work surfaces and kitchen equipment:
  - Use separate cutting boards for cooked foods and raw foods. Cut on plastic or glass cutting boards when cutting raw meat and poultry. (Wooden boards used exclusively for raw meat and poultry are acceptable; use a different board for cutting other foods, such as produce or bread.)
  - Wash cutting boards after each use in hot, soapy water; rinse and air dry or pat dry with fresh paper towels. Non-porous acrylic, plastic, or glass boards and solid wood boards can be washed in the dishwasher (laminated boards may crack and split).
  - Sanitize wooden or plastic cutting boards weekly with a solution of one part household bleach to ten parts water. Flood the surface with the solution and allow it to stand for several minutes, then rinse and air dry or pat dry with fresh paper towels. (Alternatively, use a commercial sanitizing agent and follow the directions on the product.)
  - Keep appliances free of food particles, including the microwave oven, toaster, can opener, and blender and mixer blades. Remove blender blades and the bottom ring when washing the blender container. Use a bleach solution of one part household bleach to ten parts water to sanitize these items.
  - Keep counter and kitchen surfaces free of food particles. Clean regularly with a solution of one part household bleach to ten parts water.

- Sink area:
  - Keep soap available for hand washing.
  - Use paper towels for drying hands.
  - Replace dishcloths and dish towels daily.
  - Replace sponges at least weekly.

- Sanitize sponges daily in a solution of one part household bleach to ten parts water. Or use paper towels instead of sponges while your immune system may be compromised.
- Do not store food supplies under the kitchen sink. Do not store chemicals and cleaning solutions near or over food supplies.
- Use liquid dish soap when hand washing dishes, pans, and utensils.
- Air dry dishes instead of towel-drying them.

Refrigerator/freezer:
- Keep the refrigerator clean: Clean up spills immediately, discard food scraps, and sanitize shelves and doors regularly with a solution of one part household bleach to ten parts water.
- Keep refrigerator temperature between 34 and 40 degrees F.
- Keep freezer temperature below five degrees F.
- Cool hot foods, uncovered, in the refrigerator in shallow containers; cover storage containers tightly after cooling. Freeze what you do not plan to use within the next two to three days.
- Throw away all refrigerated, cooked leftovers after 72 hours (date foods to keep track of how old the leftovers are).
- Throw out eggs with cracked shells.
- Throw out foods older than their "use by" expiration dates.
- Throw out entire food packages or containers with any mold present, including yogurt, cheese, cottage cheese, fruit, vegetables, jelly, and bread and pastry products.
- Throw out freezer-burned foods.

Cupboards/pantry:
- Throw out without tasting or opening any can with a bulge, leak, crack, or deep indentation in the seam area.
- Rotate food stock so older items are used first. Do not use foods older than their "use by" expiration dates.
- Keep food storage areas clean and monitor for signs of insect or rodent contamination.
- Review the processing used in preparing home-canned foods to be sure it was appropriate for the acidity of the food, size of the bottle, and elevation above sea level. Look for mold and leaks. Check seals. If you suspect a home-canned food may not have been processed properly

(for example, if the lid bulges, or if the food has any bad odor or unusual characteristics after opening), throw it away. Use home canned foods within one year of canning, as chemical changes may occur.

FOOD SAFETY OUTSIDE THE HOME

It's easier to control bacteria and other organisms at home than when you're in other environments. But you can keep an eye on food safety by following these tips:

- Grocery shopping:
  - Shop for shelf-stable items first, such as canned and boxed foods.
  - Check "sell by" and "use by" dates on dairy products, eggs, cereals, canned foods, and other goods. Purchase only the freshest products.
  - Check the packaging and "use by" dates on fresh meats, poultry, and seafood. Do not purchase any products that are out of date.
  - Reject damaged, swollen, rusted, or deeply dented cans. Make sure that packaged and boxed foods are properly sealed.
  - Select unblemished fruits and vegetables that look and smell fresh. Avoid wilted produce.
  - Avoid delicatessen foods.
  - In the bakery, avoid unrefrigerated cream- and custard-containing desserts and pastries.
  - Avoid foods from self-serve or bulk containers.
  - Resist trying free food samples.
  - Reject cracked or unrefrigerated eggs.
  - Select frozen and refrigerated foods last when shopping, especially during the summer months.
  - Ask that meat, poultry, and fish be placed in separate bags from fresh produce at the checkout stand.
  - Refrigerate or freeze perishables promptly, and never leave perishables in a hot car.
- Dining out:
  - Eat early to avoid crowds.
  - Ask that fresh food be prepared in fast food restaurants.
  - Ask if fruit juices are pasteurized and do not drink unpasteurized juice.
  - Avoid raw fruits and vegetables; eat these items at home where you can wash them thoroughly.

Avoiding Germs in Public Places

Stay away from salad bars and buffets where people serve themselves. Wash your hands often and use a paper towel to open the door when leaving the restroom. Don't touch your eyes, ears, nose, or mouth—this gets germs into your system.

—Tracy and Kris

- Request single-serving condiment packages and avoid self-serve bulk condiment containers. Do not eat salsa or other condiments that are unrefrigerated and used by multiple people at a restaurant.
- Avoid salad bars, delicatessens, buffets and smorgasbords, potlucks, and sidewalk vendors. These are high-risk food sources due to potentially improper food storage or holding temperature and poor hygiene by those handling the food.
- Consider the general condition of the restaurant before eating there. Are the plates, glasses, and utensils clean? Are the restrooms clean and stocked with soap and paper towels? The cleanliness of the restaurant itself may indicate the cleanliness and care involved in preparing the food.

Nutrition Suggestions for People with Weakened Immune Systems

Some foods can harbor high levels of bacteria. For example, *everyone* should avoid the following foods, whether they have a strong or weakened immune system:

- uncooked vegetable sprouts (all types, including alfalfa, radish, broccoli, mung bean, etc.) due to a high risk of contamination with *Salmonella* and *E. coli*
- raw or runny eggs, including non-pasteurized eggnog, uncooked Caesar salad dressing, and unbaked meringues to avoid bacteria (substitute frozen pasteurized eggs or powdered egg whites for raw eggs in recipes for uncooked foods)
- unpasteurized fruit and vegetable juice (unless prepared at home with washed produce)
- undercooked ground meat and poultry

Your white blood count may drop to a level that is dangerous seven to 14 days after chemotherapy. You may be at higher risk of infections at this time and may need to avoid some foods that are likely to harbor high levels of bacteria, including unwashed fruits or vegetables, unpasteurized juices, and raw or undercooked fish, meats, and eggs (see *Recommended Minimum Cooking Temperatures* on page 138).

Your doctor can tell you your current neutrophil count (neutrophils are a type of white blood cell important for fighting infection). Consider avoiding the

Go Easy on Vitamin E

Some people in cancer treatment take vitamin E supplements. Proponents claim vitamin E plays a role in protecting the body against cancer by strengthening the immune system. Some physicians believe the vitamin can also increase the effectiveness of some drugs used in chemotherapy, such as doxorubicin and 5-fluorouracil (5-FU), and reduce some of the side effects of radiation therapy. However, others believe high doses of vitamin E might interfere with the effectiveness of radiation therapy and chemotherapy. These claims are currently under investigation.

foods listed below when your immune system is extremely weak, such as when your neutrophil count falls below 1000 per microliter:

- raw and undercooked meat (including game), fish, shellfish, poultry, eggs, hot dogs, luncheon and "deli" meats, tofu, sausage, and bacon
- uncooked foods containing raw eggs, such as hollandaise sauce, raw cookie dough, or homemade mayonnaise (liquid pasteurized egg product may be used in recipes that call for raw eggs)
- raw or lightly cooked fish, shellfish, lox, sushi, or sashimi
- unpasteurized milk and dairy products (Note: you *may* eat products made from pasteurized milk, including grade A milk, hard cheeses, processed cheeses, cream cheese, cottage cheese, and yogurt.)
- soft cheeses such as feta, Brie, Camembert, blue-veined (Roquefort, Stilton, Gorgonzola, and blue), or Mexican-style cheese (such as queso blanco fresco)
- salad dressings and salsas that are not shelf-stable ("shelf stable" refers to unopened canned, bottled, or packaged food products that can be stored at room temperature before opening; the container may require refrigeration after opening)
- unwashed raw vegetables and fruits and those with visible mold
- raw honey (instead, select commercial grade A or heat-treated honey)
- "sun" tea (instead, make tea with boiling water, using commercially packaged teabags)
- unpasteurized beer
- uncooked brewer's yeast

What to Eat When Your White Blood Cell Count is Low

	Recommended	Foods that May Cause Distress
High Protein	• Well-cooked bacon, beef, chicken, fish, ham, hot dogs, lamb, pork, sausage, veal; canned fish; well-cooked pasteurized eggs or egg custard; cream, cottage, or processed cheeses; pasteurized yogurt; cooked homemade, canned, dehydrated, frozen soups	• Meat or fish salads with raw vegetables; raw fish and shellfish, such as sushi and oysters; raw or rare meats, such as steak tartare; raw or soft cooked eggs (includes "over easy," poached, soft boiled, and "sunny side up" eggs, as well as Caesar salad, homemade eggnog made with raw eggs, and raw cookie dough); cold, uncooked soups
Breads, Cereals, Rice, and Pasta	• All breads, bagels, muffins, rolls, and cereals without dried fruits, nuts, or seeds; crackers, French toast, noodles, pancakes, pasta, potatoes, and rice	• Macaroni or pasta salad or potato salad made with raw vegetables; breads or cereals with dried fruits, nuts, or seeds
Fruits and Vegetables	• Peeled thick-skinned, unblemished fruit (banana, citrus fruit, melon), peeled apples, canned fruits, cooked dried fruits; well-cooked fresh, frozen, or canned vegetables	• All other fresh or dried fruits; raw vegetables
Beverages, Desserts, and Miscellaneous	• Processed fruit juice, pasteurized milk, instant breakfast, homemade milkshakes, nondairy creamer, soda, coffee, tea, commercial liquid nutritional supplements • Fruit pies; cakes and cookies without nuts; flavored gelatin; commercial ice cream, sherbet, popsicles; pretzels, chips • Butter, margarine, cooked gravies, mayonnaise, salad dressing, vegetable oils; plain peanut butter • Salt, pepper, herbs, spices, or honey (may be added to foods only during the cooking process) • Sugar, jam, jelly, preserves, syrup, molasses, mustard, catsup; candy, chocolate; pickles, relish, olives	• Fresh-squeezed fruit juice; unpasteurized fruit juice, unpasteurized beer and wine; noncommercial ice cream, sherbet, or popsicles; popcorn • Fresh blue or Roquefort cheeses and salad dressings; Brie, Camembert, and other unpasteurized cheeses • Raw or roasted nuts; salt, pepper, herbs, spices, or honey added after cooking

People sometimes confuse low *red* blood cell counts with low *white* blood cell counts. Iron supplements won't help raise levels of white blood cells the way they increase red blood cells—there's no known supplement that can increase the white blood cell count. Of the micronutrients, zinc, selenium, iron, copper, vitamins A, C, E, and B6, and folic acid have important influences on immune responses. The best ways to make sure to get enough vitamins and minerals without harming your body with too much is by taking a daily multivitamin/mineral supplement and talking to your health care team about an optimal plan for you.

Improving Immunity in Other Ways

Now that you know how to protect yourself against bacteria and organisms that could make you ill during treatment, and you know what to eat and what to avoid, how can you improve your immune system in other ways? You may hear about ways people with cancer try to improve their immune systems. Others may promote fasting to build up the immune system. But fasting and avoiding taking in nutrients actually causes the immune system to suffer because the cells involved in providing an immune response need nutrients to run properly. (For more about fasting, see page 88 of chapter 6.) Here are some medically sound suggestions that may help improve your immune system.

COPE WITH STRESS

Being diagnosed with cancer, making decisions about treatment options, and facing uncertainties are all very stressful. Research has shown that some people with cancer experience higher-than-average levels of stress. These people tend to be at higher risk for infection. The relationship of psychological factors to infection, however, is not clearly understood. Long periods of stress or depression can lead to poor nutrition that can weaken the immune system and contribute to infection. Research also suggests that emotional stress can affect the body's hormones which, in turn, can influence the immune system. Lack of sleep, loneliness, or depression can add to stress.

Take some time for yourself, relaxing and breathing deeply. Light exercise may help you cope as well. See page 131 of chapter 9 for more information about ways to cope with stress.

National Institute of Health to Study Echinacea

Some people in cancer treatment take Echinacea supplements in an attempt to improve their immunity. Echinacea is an herb that allegedly improves the body's immune system by stimulating the activity of macrophages (immune system cells that attack and consume invading organisms), which can attack cancer cells. Some claim that the herb stimulates the anticancer activity of natural killer cells (a type of white blood cell) and therefore could be used as a supplement to chemotherapy or radiation therapy.

The National Institute of Environmental Health Sciences (NIEHS) and the Office of Dietary Supplements (ODS), components of the National Institutes of Health (NIH), have announced a five-year, $6 million grant to establish a research center to study Echinacea as well as Hypericum (St. John's wort). The goal is to learn about the effects of these potentially powerful supplements on human health.

There is currently insufficient reliable evidence to determine whether Echinacea increases resistance to cancer or alleviates the immune suppression resulting from chemotherapy.

UP AND AT 'EM

Exercise helps your immune system fight off infections, but it may also help prevent illnesses like heart disease, osteoporosis, and cancer.

Physical activity may improve your immune system by stimulating antibodies and white blood cells to move through the body more quickly than normal. Faster-moving antibodies or white blood cells could find illnesses sooner. Blood circulating more quickly may also cause the hormones that alert immune cells to bacteria or viruses to be released. And a temporarily raised body temperature may stop bacteria from growing, helping the body stave off infections—along the lines of a fever.

Exercise also prevents many stress-related hormones from being sent through the body. Stress can contribute to illness, so physical activity could minimize its effects.

Although the way exercise improves your immunity to certain illnesses isn't known for sure, being physically active helps your health in other ways—by preventing diseases like heart disease and osteoporosis, for example.

People who already exercise regularly shouldn't develop an intense workout program in the hopes of increasing immunity benefits. And before you begin a physical activity regimen for the first time, talk to your health care team. The level of activity appropriate for you depends on where you are in the course of treatment, the types of treatment you are receiving, and your general health. Your doctor and physical therapist can advise you about the level of activity that would help you most.

MEDICATIONS THAT MAY HELP

The medication filgrastim (Neupogen) is similar to a substance made by the body that stimulates the bone marrow to make more neutrophils (white blood cells) and makes them work better.

Filgrastim can be injected under the skin—the person with cancer or a family member can be taught to give the injections—or can be given intravenously. It is given at least 24 hours after chemotherapy and for up to two weeks or until the neutrophils in the blood have reached a certain level. It isn't given more than 24 hours before chemotherapy. One side effect of filgrastim is pain in the bones, which can easily be controlled. Now a long-acting form of filgrastim called peg-filgrastim (Neulasta) is available that only needs to be given once with each chemotherapy cycle.

Your blood counts will be monitored twice weekly during treatment to determine the drugs' effect on your neutrophil count.

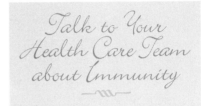

Talk to Your Health Care Team about Immunity

If the doctor tells you your immunity will be down during chemotherapy, believe it. Right after I started chemo I got strep throat...yuck! But after I had filgrastim (Neupogen) shots [used to increase white blood cells after chemotherapy] I was fine for the next six months!

Ask your pharmacist to call your insurance company and speak to a live person if there's a question about coverage—they may cover these expensive shots after all.

—Karen

Chapter 11

"*I want to stay hydrated.*"

WATER IS AS CRUCIAL TO OUR BODIES as protein, carbohydrates, fats, and vitamins and minerals. Our bodies are made up of mostly water, and we need water to survive. Every cell in the body contains water. Between 50 and 65 percent of an adult's body is made up of water.

When this fluid is balanced, it is spread throughout the proper places in the body and helps each organ function, as well as helping with crucial processes like the digestion of food, the regulation of body temperature, and creation of new tissue. Because the human body can tolerate only moderate changes in fluid balance, changes in that balance affect the way a person feels. Swelling indicates that the body is retaining too much water. Dehydration indicates that the body lacks adequate amounts of fluid or the right amount of fluid is not in the right body places.

Staying Hydrated

Hydration is essential during treatment. After treatment, water and fluids continue to be important. Continuing to stay hydrated in the long-term is important for overall health.

Experts tell us that drinking eight to 12 eight-ounce glasses (two to three quarts) of liquid a day will help keep us hydrated. It's up to us to replenish the water our bodies lose each day, but this number is somewhat arbitrary—

researchers don't know exactly how it started. Drinking plenty of water and other liquids will help your body function properly. If you have side effects like vomiting or diarrhea, you'll need to take in more liquids than normal. Talk to your health care team about hydration guidelines that make the most sense for you.

Water, pasteurized 100 percent fruit juices, milk, and broth are good choices. Caffeinated drinks add to your water supply, but as diuretics they flush more water out of the system than other choices, so don't rely on caffeinated coffee, sodas, and teas as the sole sources of your eight to 12 glasses. Liquid in your food also counts toward the total amount, and some fruits and vegetables are made up of 90 percent water. Soup, flavored ice pops, flavored ices, and gelatins also contain high percentages of water.

If you don't enjoy drinking plain water, try adding other flavors such as lemon, lime, or orange slices, or add fruit juice to give it a refreshing flavor. You may not become thirsty until after your body has lost precious water, and then you need to drink more to catch up. Keep a glass or bottle of water nearby so you're reminded to sip throughout the day, while working, reading, or watching TV.

How do you know when you're getting enough water to sustain your body? One simple way to tell is the urine test. When your urine is a pale color, you're likely getting enough water into your system; if it's dark-colored and concentrated, try upping your intake of water and other liquids. (Multivitamin/mineral supplements can darken your urine.)

Water Safety Guidelines

Drinking enough water is important during cancer treatment, and relying on safe water sources is essential when your immune system is suppressed, such as during chemotherapy treatment.

The *Water Safety Guidelines*, *Safe Water Sources*, and *Water Filters* information that follows is from *A Guide to*

Ways to Stay Hydrated

I found it very difficult to drink water, but was able to drink ginger ale and non-acidic fruit juices, particularly apple juice.

—Ling

Keep a small bottle of water handy at all times. Bottles fit in purses, packs, book bags, beverage holders in cars—just about anywhere! It's very important to stay hydrated.

—Jill

Drinking enough water daily was difficult for me until I devised this plan: Every night before going to bed I fill three 20-ounce water bottles and put them by the kitchen sink so throughout the day I see them and drink. When I finish one, I put it to the side so at a glance I can tell how much I have left to drink. I can also grab a bottle if I leave the house or drink it with a meal.

—Sharon

Good Nutrition During Cancer Treatment, Fourth Edition by Saundra Aker and Polly Lenssen and patient materials developed by Fred Hutchinson Cancer Research Center and the Seattle Cancer Care Alliance in Seattle, Washington; copyrighted materials.

Public water quality and treatment varies throughout the United States, so always check with your local health department and water utility to confirm the safety of household and community tap water and ice. Also keep in mind the issues below:

- tap water: Water from your home faucet is considered safe if your water source is a city water supply or is from a municipal well serving highly populated areas; this water is tested regularly for contamination.
- private and small community wells: The quality of well water from these sources cannot be guaranteed. *When your immune system is weak, using alternative approved water sources is recommended*, including: boiled water, bottled water, or distilled water (see the *Safe Water Sources* section below).
- filtration systems for well water: Most water filtration devices will not make the well water safe if the private well water or smaller community well water supply is not chlorinated.

SAFE WATER SOURCES

If your water is not from a city water or municipal well supply, you may want to rely on the following sources of water:

- boiled and distilled water: At home, you can make water safe by bringing tap water to a rolling boil for one minute. Distilled water can be made using a home distiller. After processing, the water should be stored in a clean, covered container in the refrigerator; discard water not used within 72 hours.
- bottled water: Acceptable forms of bottled water have been processed to remove organisms known to cause stomach or intestinal infection. Bottled water labels reading "well water," "artesian well water," "spring water," or "mineral water" do not guarantee that the water is safe to drink. *Bottled water labeled as one of the following is considered safe:*
  - reverse osmosis treated
  - distillation
  - filtered through an absolute 1 micron or smaller filter (NSF Standard #53 for cyst removal)

To be sure that a brand of bottled water has undergone one of the above processes, contact the International Bottled Water Association (IBWA; 800-928-3711; *http://www.bottledwater.org*). If IBWA does not have information on a specific brand, call the bottling company directly and ask about safety.

WATER FILTERS

If you install water filters on household water taps, make sure they meet the following specifications:

- The filters must be designed to remove *E. coli* and *Cryptosporidium*. Any of the following are acceptable:
  - reverse osmosis filter
  - absolute pore size of 1 micron or smaller
  - tested and certified by NSF Standard #53 for cyst removal
- The water tap filter must be installed immediately above the water tap.
- Manufacturer directions must be followed for filter maintenance and replacement.

Drinking Water after Chemotherapy

—⁓—

I tried to drink significantly more water for 24-48 hours after receiving the chemo drug doxorubicin hydrochloride (Adriamycin). You can see the medicine's reddish residue in your urine for a day or two after treatment. My medical oncologist recommended I try to "flush out" my system by drinking lots of water.

— Karen

Most water filtration devices will not make the water safe if the water supply has not been previously chlorinated. Portable water filters as well as refrigerator-dispensed water and ice machine systems may improve the taste or appearance of water, but they do not meet filtration standards. Portable water systems filter for chemical impurities, but not for bacteria. If a portable water system is used in combination with a safe water supply (to improve water flavor and remove chlorine and other impurities), change the system's filters frequently according to manufacturer's guidelines.

For a list of approved filtration systems, contact the National Sanitation Foundation International (800-673-8010; *http://www.NSF.org*: go to the section entitled "Home Water Treatment Devices").

Dehydration

Dehydration happens when the body loses too much water to work well. Symptoms can include a dry mouth, thirst, dizziness, weakness, an inability to swallow dry food, difficulty talking, dry skin or skin that "tents" when pinched, swollen, cracked, or dry tongue, fever, weight loss, putting out little or no urine, and feeling fatigued.

Severe diarrhea or vomiting can cause you to become dehydrated and cause an electrolyte imbalance. Acute and chronic pain can also lower the appetite so that you eat and drink less. Fatigue can be one of the first signs of dehydration. Using antiemetics, medications that provide relief from nausea and vomiting, can be very helpful and can boost the appetite and intake of liquid and food. (Antiemetics may have side effects, but most are less problematic than nausea and vomiting.)

Your health care team can help you deal with any underlying causes for altered hydration. Don't force yourself to eat or drink when you are nauseated or vomiting, and avoid eating for four to eight hours if you are vomiting often. Then you can start to try clear liquids. Begin with one teaspoonful every ten minutes, gradually increasing the amount to one tablespoon every 20 minutes. Work up to two tablespoons every 30 minutes.

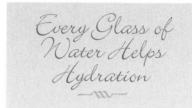

Although drinking one glass of water can sometimes feel like a huge task, it may keep you from becoming dehydrated (which happened to me more than once).

—Jen

Even small amounts of water, juices, and other clear, calorie-containing liquids throughout the day will help keep your body hydrated. You may be able to tolerate clear, cool liquids better than very hot or icy fluids, especially for an hour to a half day before treatment. But don't rely on only clear liquids for more than two days in a row. They usually don't provide the nutrients you need.

When you're eating a more typical diet of solid foods, try drinking most liquids after and/or between meals so you get enough of both liquids and solids throughout the day without becoming too full.

COPING WITH DEHYDRATION

Don't drink too much fluid at first. This can cause vomiting; instead, sip more and more fluids slowly. Good mouth care will prevent oral complications from dehydration and vomiting. (See chapter 12 for more information about oral care.)

Here are some ways to cope with dehydration:

- Suck on ice chips to relieve dry mouth.
- Drink fluids, such as water and juices.
- Try fluid-rich foods, such as fruit.
- Apply lotion to dry skin frequently.
- Treat the cause of dehydration, such as vomiting, diarrhea, or fever.
- Apply lip balm or petroleum jelly to dry lips.
- Fill a small cooler with ice and small cans of juice and keep it near you.

Liquids to Rely On

Any of the choices here add significant liquid to your diet. Your health care team can let you know if focusing on any of these foods or drinks will help you meet your nutrition goals. If you're lactose intolerant (see page 167 of chapter 12), steer clear of dairy liquids.

If vomiting or diarrhea has made you dehydrated, try small amounts of clear liquids once vomiting is under control. Begin with one teaspoonful every ten minutes, gradually increasing the amount to one tablespoon every 20 minutes. Work up to two tablespoons every 30 minutes.

When you are able to keep down clear liquids, try a full-liquid diet. Take small amounts as often as you can keep them down. If you can keep down these liquids, gradually work up to your regular diet.

Clear Liquid Diet

- bouillon
- consommé
- fruit ices without fruit pieces
- plain gelatin dessert
- strained citrus juice
- tea
- clear, fat-free broth
- cranberry/grape juice
- fruit ices without milk
- popsicles
- strained lemonade/limeade
- water
- clear carbonated beverages
- fruit-flavored drinks
- fruit punch
- sports drinks
- strained vegetable broth

Full-Liquid Diet

- all fruit juices and nectars
- carbonated beverages
- fresh or frozen plain yogurt
- ice milk
- milkshakes
- plain gelatin desserts
- small amounts of strained meat in broth or gelatin
- strained or blenderized soup
- tomato puree for cream soup
- bouillon, broth
- cheese soup
- fruit drinks
- liquid meal replacements
- pasteurized eggnog
- potatoes pureed in soup
- smooth ice cream
- soft or baked custard
- thin fruit purees
- vegetable juice
- butter/cream/oil/margarine
- coffee/tea
- fruit punch
- milk, all types
- plain cornstarch pudding
- refined/strained cooked cereal
- strained lemonade/limeade
- tomato juice
- water

Call the doctor about any of the following symptoms:

- vomiting, diarrhea, or fever lasting for more than 24 hours
- very dark urine
- inability to urinate much (or at all) for 12 hours or more
- dizziness or feeling faint when standing up
- disorientation or confusion

154

Chapter 12

"I want to cope with eating or digestion issues."

N OT EVERYONE EXPERIENCES THE EATING- AND DIGESTION-RELATED SIDE EFFECTS discussed in this chapter. If you have a friend or family member who felt ill during treatment, remember that he or she is not you. Everyone reacts differently.

Coping with Eating or Digestion Issues

Some eating and especially digestion issues may be embarrassing to talk about at first. Remember that thousands of others have experienced side effects at some point during their treatment. Your health care team's goal is to treat your cancer while helping you stay strong. Part of that mission includes helping you address how to keep nutrients in your body so they can do their job and keep you healthy. Don't be afraid to talk about your experiences and concerns in order to come up with a plan.

Digestion Challenges

If you do experience these types of challenges, remember that you may try various tactics to cope with side effects of treatment before finding the combination that helps you. There are ways to successfully deal with the basic challenges of eating and digesting food during treatment.

Acupuncture May Help Control Chemotherapy Side Effects

People with cancer receiving high-dose chemotherapy found that electroacupuncture treatments (which passes a low electrical current through acupuncture needles placed in specific points on the body) combined with antinausea medication were more effective than medication alone in controlling their chemotherapy-related vomiting, according to a study.

The treatment consisted of needles inserted in classic antiemetic (anti-vomiting) acupuncture points—in both arms over the wrist, and on the outside of both legs near the knees. A pulse generator connected to the needles provided an electrical current to the points. Treatments were always given within two hours before chemotherapy.

Newer approaches to chemotherapy have dramatically decreased the incidence of nausea and vomiting in people receiving chemotherapy. But electroacupuncture could help those who still have nausea and vomiting.

People with cancer are finding that electroacupuncture can sometimes be effective in dealing with pain, nausea, and treatment of mucositis (ulcerations or swelling in the mouth). The treatment is being provided at many cancer centers. More research is needed to find out how effective electroacupuncture is in treating nausea and vomiting for people who have cancer. Most health insurance does not cover acupuncture.

CONTROLLING NAUSEA AND VOMITING

People in cancer treatment may have nausea and vomiting, most often caused by radiation or chemotherapy treatments. If you receive chemotherapy, the type of drug you receive may or may not make you feel ill. Many of them don't cause these side effects. Some people tolerate treatment more easily than others, and you may get used to your treatment and experience few side effects.

Nausea and vomiting vary widely. Some people receiving cancer treatments may never have these symptoms. For others, just thinking about going to the treatments for cancer can cause nausea or vomiting. Frequent vomiting can be dangerous if it leads to dehydration or to choking.

Don't force yourself to eat or drink when you are nauseated or vomiting, and avoid eating for four to eight hours if you are vomiting often. After that time, start to try clear liquids. But don't rely on only clear liquids for more than two days in a row.

How to cope with nausea and vomiting. If you need to rest after eating, try sitting up or reclining with your head elevated for an hour or so. Food odors sometimes cause nausea; for more information about coping with food odors, see the *Managing Changes in Taste and Smell* section on page 179 of this chapter.

If you are receiving a cancer treatment that is likely to cause nausea and vomiting, ask your doctor about antiemetics. Generally, a person with cancer begins taking antinausea medicines before their treatment begins and continues taking them while treatment may cause vomiting. Do not wait until you are vomiting to take antiemetics; these medicines are usually meant to be taken on a regular schedule to prevent vomiting. Your health care team might give you more than one antinausea medicine since certain types work differently. Many effective antinausea medicines are available. If you continue to have nausea and vomiting while taking antiemetics, be sure to tell your doctor so he or she can provide a new medicine.

After you have stopped vomiting, be sure to take in plenty of fluids to prevent dehydration—try a liquid diet or easy-to-digest foods including clear liquids and crackers, gelatin, and plain toast. Some other tips for coping include:

- If you are in bed, lie on your side so you do not inhale or swallow vomit.
- Request that medications be prescribed in suppository form if you can't swallow.
- Take liquids in the form of ice chips or frozen juice chips that can be sucked on slowly.

Call the doctor about any of the following symptoms:

- inhalation of or swallowed vomited material
- vomiting more than three times an hour for three or more hours
- blood or material that looks like coffee grounds in your vomit
- inability to consume more than four cups of liquid or ice chips in a day or inability to eat more substantial foods for more than two days

Coping with Nausea and Vomiting

I found it very helpful to have the nurse inject the chemo drugs slowly. When they were pushed in too fast, I immediately felt nauseated and very uncomfortable.

—*Ling*

I absolutely encourage all patients and caregivers to discuss digestion problems with healthcare professionals and other patients. You may not find the right trick or medication for you on the first or even the fifth try, but keep at it, and eventually you will find the drug, food or activity that works for you.

—*Kathi*

Eat a light snack or meal on the day of chemo, but not less than two hours before treatment. I have a very sensitive stomach but followed this rule of thumb and never once vomited during treatment.

—*Jan*

- inability to take medications
- weakness or dizziness

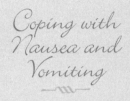

Coping with Nausea and Vomiting

Coffee seemed to worsen my nausea pretty dramatically, so I avoided it for many months. Conversely, green tea was soothing and a way to promote improved fluid intake.

Most cruciferous vegetables significantly worsened my nausea and vomiting. The mere smell of them cooking was enough to prompt vomiting, so I avoided these throughout treatment, although ordinarily I ate them regularly. Oddly enough, my mother's cabbage, ham, and cheese casserole tasted good to me, stayed down, and I was able to eat it fairly often.

However, I could not be in the house while it was being cooked; the smell caused immediate gastrointestinal distress.

— Kathi

When eating out, ask for a table as far from the kitchen as possible to avoid cooking odors.

— Norma Jean

How to eat when you have nausea and vomiting. Don't be afraid to experiment with recipes, flavorings, spices, types, and consistencies of food. Food likes and dislikes may change from day to day. Drink eight or more cups of liquid each day if you can. Drink an additional half cup to one cup of liquid for each episode of vomiting. Try sipping liquids 30 to 60 minutes after eating solid food.

When and how to eat:
- If you have nausea only between meals, eat six to eight frequent, small meals and snack at bedtime.
- Eat food cold or at room temperature to decrease its smell and taste.
- Avoid eating in a room that is warm.
- Rinse your mouth before and after meals.
- Sit up or recline with your head raised for at least an hour after eating if you need to rest.
- Suck on hard candy, such as peppermint or lemon, if there is a bad taste in your mouth.
- Try adding ginger to your diet; some research shows that ginger can relieve nausea, although studies of ginger's ability to reduce nausea and vomiting after surgery have shown mixed results.

What to eat:
- Slowly sip cold, clear liquids, like ginger ale. (Fresh ginger or ginger tea may help alleviate nausea, although not chemotherapy-induced nausea.)
- Eat fish and chicken if you develop a distaste for red meat and meat broths, which is common in people with cancer.
- Eat dry foods, such as crackers, toast, dry cereals, or bread sticks, when you wake up and every few hours during the day.
- Eat cool foods instead of hot, spicy foods.

Take It Easy

If you feel nauseous when you're anticipating a visit to the doctor, consider hypnosis or other relaxation therapies to lessen nausea. Nutrition, hypnosis, acupuncture, and guided imagery may help relieve nausea and vomiting and may also improve the effectiveness of antinausea drugs. Also consider trying the following ways of alleviating nausea:

- Rest comfortably in a quiet environment.
- Try to rest quietly for at least an hour after each meal.
- Distract yourself with soft music, a favorite television program, or company.
- Try to relax and take slow, deep breaths when you feel nauseous.
- Avoid unnecessary stimulation or excitement.
- Eat salty crackers to help settle your stomach.

- Avoid foods that are overly sweet, greasy, fried, or spicy, such as rich desserts and french fries.
- Try bland, soft, easy-to-digest foods on scheduled treatment days.
- Eat foods without a strong odor.

MANAGING CONSTIPATION

Changes in your eating habits, general weakness, postponing trips to the bathroom, and decreased physical activity can cause constipation (when the bowels move less frequently and stools become more difficult to pass). For people with cancer, constipation may be a symptom of cancer, a result of a growing tumor, or a result of cancer treatment. Dehydration and not eating enough may also contribute to constipation, as can other changes in the body, such as organ failure, a decreased ability to move, or depression, for example.

Constipation may also be a side effect of medications for cancer or cancer pain, such as pain medications, medications for anxiety and depressions, stomach antacids, diuretics, multivitamin/mineral supplements containing iron and calcium, sleep medications, or general anesthesia. Constipation can be a chemotherapy side effect. Some chemotherapy drugs may intensify an existing problem with constipation, especially for the elderly and those who are eating low-fiber diets.

What to Eat During Chemotherapy

Talk to your doctor about trying the following eating guidelines on the days you receive chemotherapy. Keep in mind, however, that this diet is not adequate in protein, calories, vitamins, and minerals. It should be followed for no more than three days. If you can't eat more foods after three days, tell your doctor.

What to Eat on the Day of Therapy When Nausea and Vomiting May Be a Problem

	Recommended	Foods that May Cause Distress
High Protein	Juice-type commercial supplements	All others
Breads, Cereals, Rice, and Pasta	Dry toast, saltines, rice	All others
Fruits and Vegetables	Apple, cranberry, and grape juice	All others
Beverages, Desserts, and Miscellaneous	Ginger ale; decaffeinated, noncarbonated drinks such as fruit punch and sports drinks; popsicles, fruit ice, sherbet; flavored gelatin; pretzels	All others

What to Eat on Other Days When Nausea and Vomiting Is a Problem

	Recommended	Foods that May Cause Distress
High Protein	Boiled, baked meat, fish, poultry; cold meat or fish salad; eggs; cream soups made with low-fat milk; low-fat luncheon meat; lean ham; nonfat yogurt	Fatty and fried meats, such as sausage, bacon; fried eggs; milkshakes (unless made with low-fat milk or ice cream)
Breads, Cereals, Rice, and Pasta	Saltines, soda crackers, bread, toast, cold cereal, English muffins, bagels, plain noodles, rice	Doughnuts, pastries, waffles, pancakes, muffins
Fruits and Vegetables	Potatoes (baked, boiled, or mashed), juices, canned or fresh fruits, vegetables as tolerated (omit if appetite is poor or nausea is severe)	Potato chips, french fries, hash browns; breaded, fried, or creamed vegetables; vegetables with strong odor
Beverages, Desserts, and Other Foods	Cold fruit drinks, decaffeinated soft drinks, iced tea, sports drinks; sherbet, fruit-flavored gelatin; angel food cake, sponge cake; vanilla wafers; pudding (made with low-fat milk); popsicles, juice bars, fruit ices; pretzels; butter or margarine in small amounts, fat-skimmed gravy; salt, cinnamon, spices as tolerated	Alcohol, coffee; pie, ice cream, rich cakes; spicy salad dressings, olives, cream, pepper, chili powder, onion, hot sauce, seasoning mixtures

©2000, American Dietetic Association. "The Clinical Guide to Oncology Nutrition: Patient Education Materials." Used with permission.

Relax When Constipated

Constipation may cause you to become anxious about your bowel movements. Try to relax, which may help you move your bowels. You may also want to try the following:

- Drink a warm or hot drink about a half hour before your usual time for a bowel movement.
- Provide privacy and quiet time when you need to have a bowel movement.
- Ask for help getting to the toilet if you need it, or for a bedside commode instead of a bedpan.

If you have had bowel surgery for your cancer, you may experience intermittent constipation or diarrhea for several months afterward.

Talk to your health care team about bowel movements that are hard, diarrhea-like stool, cramps or stomach pain, gas, expanded abdomen, vomiting or nausea, no stool movement for three days, and any other pain or discomfort.

How to cope with constipation. Keep a record of all bowel movements to help your doctor develop a plan to cope with constipation. If you are constipated, try to stimulate your bowels to move by following these tips:

- Drink plenty of fluids to keep your digestive system moving.
- Try to have a bowel movement at the same time each day to establish regularity.
- Avoid using extreme force or straining in trying to move your bowels.
- Try to eat at the same times each day.
- To lessen the amount of air you swallow while eating, try not to talk much at meals, drink without straws, and avoid chewing gum.
- Get as much light exercise as possible, including abdominal exercises in bed or moving from the bed to chair if you aren't able to walk.
- Use stool softeners or laxatives as instructed by your doctor or nurse.
- Ask your dietitian to recommend a high-calorie, high-protein, fiber-containing liquid supplement (such as Metamucil, FiberCon, Milk of Magnesia, Benefiber, or Colace) if you need more calories, protein, and fiber.

High-Fiber Foods to Choose More Often

These nutritious foods may help alleviate constipation.

	Serving Size	Dietary Fiber (grams)
Breads and Cereals		
bran cereals	½ cup	3–13
popcorn	2 cups	5
brown rice	½ cup	6
whole-wheat bread	1 slice	1–2
wheat bran, raw	¼ cup	6
Legumes		
kidney beans*	½ cup	8
navy beans*	½ cup	9
Vegetables		
broccoli*	½ cup	4
brussels sprouts*	½ cup	3
carrots	½ cup	2
corn	½ cup	5
green peas	½ cup	3
potato with skin	1 medium	3
Fruit		
apple with peel	1 medium	4
banana	1 medium	2
blueberries	½ cup	2
pear with skin	1 medium	5
prunes	3	3
orange	1 medium	3
raisins	¼ cup	3
strawberries	1 cup	3

*These foods tend to cause gas.

Call the doctor about any of the following symptoms:

- no bowel movement in three days
- blood in or around anal area or in stool
- no bowel movement within two days of taking a laxative
- persistent cramps or vomiting

How to eat when you're constipated. Stay away from foods that may cause constipation in some individuals, such as chocolates, cheese, and eggs. If you have had a bowel obstruction or bowel surgery (for example, a colostomy), don't eat a high-fiber diet. Don't use over-the-counter laxatives or enemas, especially if your white blood cell count or platelet count is low, except as instructed by your doctor. These treatments may lead to bleeding, infection, or other harmful side effects in people with cancer. Instead, try the following:

- Increase your intake of high-fiber and bulky foods, such as whole-grain breads and cereals, fresh raw or cooked fruits with skins and seeds, fresh raw vegetables, fruit juices, dried fruits, seeds, dates, apricots, prunes, popcorn, dried beans, and nuts.
- Drink more fluids when increasing dietary fiber or your constipation may become worse.
- Avoid gas-producing foods and beverages (such as cabbage, broccoli, cauliflower, cucumbers, dried beans, peas, onions, and carbonated drinks) if they become a problem.
- Drink more fluids to help prevent dehydration— eight to 12 glasses of liquid each day, if it's okay with your doctor. Try water, prune juice, fresh juices (except apple juice), and warm or hot fluids in the morning, such as teas, juices, and hot lemonade.
- Eat a breakfast that includes a hot drink and high-fiber foods.
- Caffeine may also help alleviate constipation.

COPING WITH DIARRHEA

Cancer treatments and medications can cause your bowels to move much more frequently and stools to become very loose. Diarrhea is the passage of loose or watery stools three or more times a day, with or without discomfort. It occurs when the water in the intestine is not, for some reason, reabsorbed back into the body.

Diarrhea can sometimes be caused by an overflow of intestinal liquids around stool that is lodged (impacted) in the intestine. Other causes include bacterial and viral infections; side effects of chemotherapy or radiation therapy to

Coping with Diarrhea

When I was on the chemotherapy drugs cyclophosphamide (Cytoxan) and paclitaxel (Taxol), my medical oncologist warned me I might have constipation, diarrhea, or both. I thought it was impossible, but you can have constipation and diarrhea at the same time! To ease the discomfort, I tried to avoid food that could bind me up, such as cheese and bananas. I tried to eat more fruits like raisins, grapes, prunes, etc. to keep things moving. I also used Preparation H pads after every bowel movement to keep things clean and reduce swelling.

—Karen

the abdomen; medications; surgery; anxiety; supplemental feedings containing large amounts of vitamins, minerals, and sugar; and tumor growth. Diarrhea caused by chemotherapy or radiation therapy may continue for up to three weeks after treatment and varies from person to person. Treat it early, and talk to your doctor about ongoing diarrhea.

How to cope with diarrhea. If you have diarrhea, be sure to sip fluids throughout the day to prevent dehydration, a serious potential result of diarrhea. When the diarrhea starts to improve, begin eating small amounts of low-fiber foods, such as rice, bananas, applesauce, yogurt, mashed potatoes, low-fat cottage cheese, and dry toast.

Monitor the amount and frequency of your bowel movements, and rely on some of the following tips to cope with diarrhea:

- Try a clear liquid diet (water, weak tea, apple juice, peach nectar, clear broth, popsicles, plain gelatin) as soon as diarrhea starts or when you feel that it is going to start. Clear liquids keep the bowels from working too hard and guard against its irritation.
- Eat frequent small meals.
- Eat foods that are high in pectin, like applesauce and bananas.
- Drink and eat foods that are high in potassium (such as fruit juices and nectars, sports drinks, potatoes without the skin, and bananas), an important mineral often lost through diarrhea. Potassium helps muscles function properly.
- Drink and eat foods that are high in sodium, such as soups, broths, sports drinks, crackers, and pretzels.
- If diarrhea lasts longer than two days, start a liquid diet and add low-fiber foods as tolerated.
- Drink at least a cup of liquid after each bout of diarrhea.

Call the doctor about any of the following symptoms:

- six or more loose bowel movements per day, with no improvement in two days
- blood in or around anal area or in stool

Coping with Diarrhea

Disposable, flushable wipes were a great comfort when my gut was at its worst. I carried a few in my purse in a sealable plastic bag at all times and kept containers of them in all our bathrooms throughout treatment. They provided comfort and made me feel clean, despite all those frequent trips to the restroom. The elasticized legs and waist "pull-on" diapers were the most comfortable and provided the best protection. I do not recommend the adult diapers with the side tapes if you are up and about. They were uncomfortable and weren't dependable protection in my case.

— Kathi

Pamper Yourself

Diarrhea can irritate the anal area. Be gentle and take special care of this sensitive area when you're experiencing diarrhea.

- Clean the anal area with a mild soap after each bowel movement, rinse well with warm water, and pat dry.
- Try using soothing flushable wipes instead of toilet paper when you're having diarrhea to prevent irritation.
- Inspect your anal area for red, scaly, broken skin.
- Apply a water-repellent cream, such as Vaseline or A&D ointment, to the anal area.
- Try sitz baths (bathing the hips and buttocks in a warm bath to reduce pain or discomfort in the anal area).
- Take medicine for diarrhea or skin irritation as recommended by your doctor.

- weight loss of five pounds or more after the diarrhea starts
- new abdominal cramps or pain lasting two or more days
- inability to urinate for 12 or more hours
- inability to drink any liquids for more than two days
- fever
- suddenly puffy or bloated abdomen
- constipation for several days accompanied by a small amount of diarrhea or oozing of fecal material, suggesting fecal impaction
- continuing or worsening diarrhea or stools that have an unusual odor or color

How to eat when you have diarrhea. Using tobacco products, drinking caffeinated, alcoholic, or carbonated beverages, and eating very hot or very cold foods may irritate your digestive tract. Don't consume only clear liquids for more than two days in a row without a doctor's supervision, since you don't get many nutrients from this diet. Other foods that may stimulate or irritate the digestive tract include the following:

- high-fat foods such as fried, greasy, and rich foods, which can promote diarrhea

Food List: How to Eat to Alleviate Diarrhea

	Recommended	Foods that May Cause Distress
Protein	Baked or broiled beef, pork, chicken, turkey, veal, fish, eggs, milk, cheese; yogurt	
Breads, Cereals, Rice, and Pasta	Bread and rolls make from refined, white flour; pasta; converted or instant rice; refined cereals such as farina, Cream of Wheat, Cream of Rice, oatmeal, cornflakes; pancakes; waffles, cornbread; muffins; graham crackers	Whole-grain breads and cereals such as whole-wheat and rye bread; bran; shredded wheat; granola; wild rice
Fruits and Vegetables	Soups made with allowed vegetables; cooked asparagus tips, beets, carrots, peeled zucchini, mushrooms, celery, tomato paste, tomato puree, tomato sauce; baked potato without skin; canned, frozen, or fresh fruit	Fresh, unpeeled fruit; pears; melon; all other vegetables
Beverages, Desserts, and Other Foods	Butter; margarine; mayonnaise; salad dressing; vegetable oil; cake; cookies; flavored gelatin desserts; sherbet; fruit pie made with allowed fruit; decaffeinated beverages; salt pepper, spices, and gravy as tolerated	Desserts with nuts; coconut; dried fruit; chocolate; licorice; pickles; popcorn; foods with a lot of pepper, chili seasoning, or taco seasoning; hot sauces

©2000, American Dietetic Association. "The Clinical Guide to Oncology Nutrition: Patient Education Materials." Used with permission.

- foods that cause gas (such as gas-forming vegetables and chewing gum) and carbonated beverages (you may be able to drink carbonated beverages if you leave them open for at least ten minutes before drinking)
- nuts, raw fruits or vegetables, whole-grain breads, and cereals or products made with bran
- milk and milk products (including creamed soups, puddings, and milkshakes)
- strong spices and herbs

Chemotherapy, radiation to the abdomen, antibiotics, or treatments that affect the gastrointestinal tract may make you lactose intolerant, which means that your body isn't producing enough of the enzyme lactase to break down the milk sugar lactose.

When lactose isn't broken down, it remains in the intestine, where the body directs water to try to dilute it and where bacteria ferment the lactose. This fluid retention and fermentation can cause diarrhea, gas, and cramping. These symptoms disappear after treatment sessions are over or when the digestive system has healed.

How to cope with lactose intolerance. You can monitor your intake of lactose to figure out the level you can tolerate without having difficulty. If the lactose intolerance continues, your health care team may recommend a low-lactose or lactose-free diet. If this diet is recommended for you, keep an eye on food ingredient lists—lactose is not only found where milk is a primary ingredient; it's also often used to sweeten foods.

If you're unable to eat dairy products without digestive distress and are concerned about getting enough calcium in your diet, try to eat more of the following calcium-rich foods:

- kelp
- leafy green vegetables such as broccoli and greens
- nuts
- seeds
- beans
- tofu (prepared with calcium)
- dried figs
- oysters
- canned fish that still has bones, such as sardines and salmon
- foods labeled as calcium-fortified, such as juice, crackers, and cereal

What to eat when you're lactose intolerant. Foods that include whey, casein, and nonfat milk solids may contribute to digestive challenges; try small portions of them to find out your level of tolerance. Gum, peppermint, butterscotch, and artificial sweeteners may also include lactose. Lactose is sometimes also found as a filler in some tablet medications, so check the ingredients of any of these types of medicines you're taking often and speak to your health care team about other options if problems persist.

Foods that contain lactose and should be avoided can include the following:

- Beverages:
  - milk (liquid or dry, including skim, dried, evaporated, or condensed and acidophilus milk)
  - malted milk
  - hot chocolate, some cocoas and instant coffees, and other powdered drinks
  - powdered coffee creamer

- Dairy:
  - omelets or soufflés made using milk, cheese, or chocolate
  - cheeses, except those naturally aged

- Breads and cereals:
  - breads, dry cereals, and hot cereals
  - prepared mixes for muffins, waffles, pancakes, and biscuits

- Desserts:
  - ice cream and sherbet
  - custards and puddings
  - chocolate
  - pie crust made using margarine or butter
  - desserts with cream fillings

- Meats, fruits, and vegetables:
  - creamed vegetables and meat
  - meats and vegetables to which lactose is added during processing including peas or instant potatoes
  - canned or frozen fruit processed with lactose

- Sauces and sides:
  - gravies
  - creamy soups, sauces, dressings, and dips
  - sour cream
  - other prepared products that contain dry milk solids

- Fats:
  - margarine or butter
  - cream
  - cream cheese
  - peanut butter with milk solids

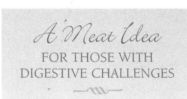

A Meat Idea

FOR THOSE WITH
DIGESTIVE CHALLENGES

While my husband was on chemotherapy, he ate lamb cuts (chops, roast, etc.) without experiencing digestive side effects. He found this to be the most agreeable meat to eat.

—Florence

Keep in mind the following lactose-free and other options:

- Soy or rice milks, which come in flavors like chocolate and vanilla as well as regular, are an alternative to dairy milks. They often taste best when very cold. (Soy and rice milk don't supply the same nutrients as cow milk. But fortified soy or rice milk can be good substitutes, especially when you're receiving necessary protein and fat in other areas of your diet.)
- Lactaid products are milk products with the enzyme lactase already added to help with digestion.
- You can often find other milk substitutes at stores that carry health food products. Choose high-calorie, full-fat substitutes over low-calorie, low-fat options so your body gets all of the nutrients it needs.
- Imitation sour cream, non-dairy whipped topping, and soy cheese are good lactose-free options.
- You may be able to tolerate cultured dairy products such as buttermilk, yogurt, and some cheeses; they will have less lactose and the active cultures will help you to digest it.
- Use a commercial lactase enzyme when cooking with milk.

You may want to speak to your doctor, nurse, or dietitian about tablets that contain the lactase enzyme and can help in the digestion of milk products. According to their directions, add the tablets to dairy before eating; they must be in contact with the dairy product for a while before you eat the dairy in order to break down lactose. This should make the digestion process easier without reducing the nutritional value of the dairy food.

You will probably eventually be able to add foods containing lactose back into your diet in small amounts.

Eating and Swallowing Challenges

Oral complications are common in people with cancer, especially those with head and neck cancer. This section describes oral complications caused by chemotherapy and radiation therapy, how to prevent them when possible, and ways of handling them if they arise.

When cancer treatment is over, good dental hygiene like brushing and flossing to remove plaque will help minimize the oral effects of cancer treatment such as swelling in the mouth. Flavored oral products can irritate fragile tissue or burn the gums and mouth, and products that contain alcohol can hurt your mouth. Try a mild toothpaste, like a children's toothpaste.

Caring for Your Mouth and Throat When You Have Difficulty Eating and Swallowing

	Sore Mouth or Throat	Mouth Sores	Bleeding in Mouth	Dry Mouth	Difficulty Swallowing
Clean or rinse your teeth (including dentures) and mouth 30 minutes after eating and every four hours.	X	X	X	X	
Brush the teeth using a soft nylon-bristle toothbrush and a non-abrasive toothpaste or baking soda solution. Rinse toothbrush well after each use and store in a cool, dry place.	X	X	X	X	X
Use water-soluble lubricating jelly to moisturize the mouth.	X				
Clean your mouth gently with a soft toothbrush, toothette (a foam swab on a stick), or gauze dipped in saltwater.	X	X	X	X	
Use petroleum jelly or lip balm to moisten lips.		X		X	
Check your mouth twice a day using a small flashlight and a padded tongue blade; if you wear dentures, remove them first.		X			
Report any changes in appearance, taste, or feeling in your mouth to your doctor or nurse.		X			
Use a cool mist humidifier to moisten room air, especially at night. (Be sure to keep the humidifier clean to avoid spreading bacteria or mold in the air.)				X	X
Ask your doctor or pharmacist about artificial saliva.				X	X
Drink at least six to eight cups of fluids daily, with approval from your doctor.	X	X	X	X	X
Try sipping warm tea to soothe your mouth and throat.		X			
Ask your pharmacist about Miracle Mouthwash, a solution of Maalox, viscous lidocaine (a prescription local anesthetic or pain reliever), and Benadryl elixir that may help numb and soothe the mouth.	X	X			

SOOTHING A SORE MOUTH OR THROAT

One of the most common oral problems occurring after chemotherapy and radiation therapy to the neck or chest area is an inflammation of the mucous membranes in the mouth. You may develop mucositis, or swelling of the mouth, seven to 10 days after treatment. It will heal on its own in two to four weeks if there isn't an infection. How to treat it depends on how severe it is and your white blood cell count.

How to cope with a sore or irritated mouth and throat. Eating a well-balanced diet, maintaining good oral hygiene, and finding any oral problems early can help minimize possible problems. If your health care team advises you that your treatment has a high possibility of oral challenges, see a dentist or hygienist (one who knows about the oral complications of cancer treatment before chemotherapy or radiation therapy to the head and neck) at least a month before treatment so any dental work can heal before treatment.

COPING WITH MOUTH SORES

Mouth sores are like little cuts or ulcers in the mouth that may bleed. The sores may be very red, or they may have small white patches in the middle. Open sores in the mouth occur in many people receiving chemotherapy, and about half of the people who undergo chemotherapy have severe lesions that require medical treatment, including changes in cancer medication.

Chemotherapy can cause mouth sores. If that's the case, they typically occur one to two weeks after treatment. They can also be caused by radiation therapy to the head and neck area or by infection, dehydration, poor mouth care, or lack of protein in the diet. With proper care, mouth sores can heal in about two to four weeks.

Mouth sores can cause a combination of the following: red, shiny, or swollen mouth and gums, blood in the mouth, small ulcers or sores in the mouth, on the gums, or

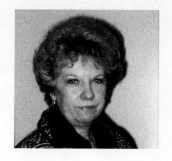

What to Eat When Your Throat or Mouth is Sore

	Recommended	Foods that May Cause Distress
High Protein	Ground, chopped, or blenderized meats, poultry, or fish; casseroles; egg, cheese, and bean dishes; milkshakes, yogurt, and commercial liquid nutritional supplements	Whole meats, poultry, fish, dry meats
Breads, Cereals, Rice, and Pasta	Moistened breads, cooked cereals, cold cereal soaked in milk, pasta and rice in sauce	Dry toast, hard rolls, dry crackers, English muffins, bagels
Fruits and Vegetables	Cooked or blenderized fruits; fruits and vegetables	Fresh fruits and vegetables (unless very ripe, soft, and juicy, such as applesauce, bananas, and watermelon); citrus fruit, pineapple, and other acidic fruit, pickled fruit; raw and pickled fruits and vegetables
Beverages, Desserts, and Miscellaneous	Fruit nectars, flavored gelatin, ice cream, sherbet, pudding; butter, margarine, and vegetable oils	Carbonated beverages; cookies and cakes unless soaked in milk; crunchy snacks such as pretzels and chips; vinegar; condiments such as pepper, pepper sauces, chili powder, cloves, nutmeg, salsa

©2000, American Dietetic Association. "The Clinical Guide to Oncology Nutrition: Patient Education Materials." Used with permission.

on the tongue, white or yellow film in the mouth, pain in the mouth, mouth dryness, mild burning, or increased sensitivity to hot and cold foods, soft, whitish patches or pus in the mouth, or increased mucus in the mouth.

How to cope with mouth sores. Mouth sores can make eating regularly painful, and your favorite foods may irritate a sensitive mouth. Talk to the doctor or cancer care team about using medication to treat mouth sores. If mouth pain is severe or interferes with eating, ask your doctor to recommend a medicine that can be swished and swallowed 15 minutes before meals or painted on the painful areas with a cotton swab before meals.

How to Eat When You Have Difficulty Eating or Swallowing

	Sore Mouth or Throat	Mouth Sores	Bleeding in Mouth	Dry Mouth	Difficulty Swallowing
Avoid tart, acidic, or salty foods such as pickled and vinegary foods, citrus fruits, tomato-based foods, some canned broths, and irritating spices, seasonings and condiments such as pepper, chili powder, cloves, nutmeg, pepper sauces, and horseradish.	X	X	X	X	X
Avoid citrus fruit juices (grapefruit, orange, lemon, and lime) and carbonated beverages.	X	X	X	X	X
Avoid rough-textured foods, such as dry toast, pretzels, granola, and raw fruits and vegetables.	X	X	X	X	X
Avoid foods that need a lot of chewing, such as meats, chewy candy, or raw whole vegetables.				X	X
Avoid very hot or very cold foods .	X	X	X	X	X
Stay away from alcohol, caffeine, and tobacco.	X	X	X	X	X
Avoid irritating spices such as chili powder, cloves, curry, hot sauces, nutmeg, and pepper.	X	X	X	X	X
Eat soft, bland, creamy foods high in calories and protein, such as cream soups, cheeses, mashed potatoes, yogurt, eggs, custards, puddings, cooked cereals, ice cream, casseroles, gravies, syrups, milkshakes, and commercial liquid food supplements.	X	X	X	X	X
Blend and moisten dry or solid foods with gravies, yogurt, milk, broth, creams, butter, or margarine.	X			X	X
Drink through a straw.		X	X	X	
Avoid hot drinks. (Heat dilates blood vessels and increases bleeding.)				X	
Try chilled foods and fluids, such as popsicles, apple-sauce, yogurt, frozen yogurt, sherbet, and ice cream.	X	X	X	X	
Eat six to eight small meals a day.					X

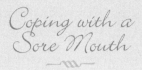
To promote healing, ask your doctor about using Maalox or Milk of Magnesia. Allow the medicine to settle and separate, pour off the liquid top of the solution, and swab the paste part onto the sore area with a cotton swab. Rinse after about 20 minutes.

Call the doctor about any of the following symptoms:

- redness or shininess in mouth that lasts for more than 48 hours
- bleeding gums
- cuts or sores in the mouth
- temperature of 100.5 degrees F or higher
- white patches on the tongue or on the inside of the mouth

CONTROLLING BLEEDING IN THE MOUTH

Bleeding in the mouth is generally caused by mouth sores, gum (periodontal) disease, or by a decrease in the number of platelets (a blood component responsible for blood clotting). This is usually a temporary problem. Platelets can decrease as a side effect of radiation therapy, chemotherapy, or because of disease. A person with decreased platelets bleeds easily; an everyday action such as brushing teeth can result in bleeding. Side effects of chemotherapy or radiation therapy can cause dryness of the lining of the mouth or the formation of small mouth ulcers that result in bleeding.

Bleeding in the mouth can take the form of blood or bruises in mouth (or on the gums or tongue), a rash or bright red pinpoint-sized dots on the tongue, under the tongue, on the roof of mouth, and/or on the inside of the cheeks.

How to cope with bleeding in the mouth. Call the doctor about any of the following symptoms:

- when you bleed from mouth for the first time
- if bleeding continues for more than a half hour
- if you vomit blood
- if you feel light-headed

Cleaning and Moisturizing the Mouth

Rinsing your mouth often with one of the following mixtures will help keep it clean and soothed:

- sterile water
- one teaspoon of baking soda in two cups of water
- ½ teaspoon of salt in one quart of water
- one part hydrogen peroxide in three parts water; mix right before use and hold in mouth for one and a half minutes (use for only one or two days because it may keep mouth sores from healing.)

Rinsing often cleans and moistens the tissues, prevents crusting, and soothes sore gums and tissues. Frequent rinsing prevents particles and bacteria from collecting in the mouth. A salt and baking soda solution neutralizes acids and dissolves thick saliva.

MANAGING A DRY MOUTH OR THICK SALIVA

Radiation therapy to the head and neck may injure the glands that produce saliva, the inside of the mouth, the muscles of the jaw and neck, and/or the jaw bones. This can cause dry mouth, also called xerostomia.

Dry mouth occurs when there is not enough saliva in the mouth. Breathing through the mouth can cause it, as can some medications or dehydration. If you have a dry mouth or thick saliva, you might experience dried, flaky, whitish-colored saliva in and around the mouth, thick, stringy saliva that stays attached to the lips when you open your mouth, or constant debris stuck to the teeth, tongue, and gums.

How to cope with a dry mouth or thick saliva. If you have a dry mouth or thick saliva, drink plenty of fluids throughout the day and incorporate moist foods into your diet as much as possible. Suck on sugar-free lollipops, sour lemon drops, or frozen grapes to get saliva going.

Call the doctor about any of the following symptoms:

- a dry mouth for more than three days
- dry, cracked lips or mouth sores
- difficulty breathing

What to Eat When You Have a Dry Mouth

	Recommended	Foods that May Cause Distress
High Protein	Meats, poultry, and fish in sauces and gravies, casseroles, soups, and stews	Dry meats, poultry, and fish without sauces
Breads, Cereals, Rice, and Pasta	Bread, soft rolls; cooked and cold cereals, cereal with milk; rice soaked in gravy, sauce, broth, or milk	Dry breads, hard rolls, pasta, rice, pretzels, chips, cereal
Fruits and Vegetables	Canned and fresh fruits that have a lot of moisture, such as oranges and peaches; vegetables in sauce	Bananas, dried fruit, vegetables unless in a sauce or with a high moisture content
Beverages, Desserts, and Miscellaneous	Club soda, hot tea with lemon, fruit-ades, diluted juices, sports drinks, commercial liquid nutrition supplements, homemade milkshakes; ice cream, sherbet, pudding; butter, margarine, salad dressing; sour cream, half-and-half	Cookies, cake, pie, unless soaked in milk

Coping with Swallowing Problems

When dining out, always ask for water with your meal; it helps alleviate swallowing difficulties.
— *Louise*

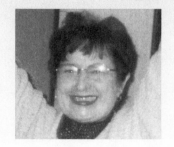

MAKING IT EASIER TO SWALLOW

People with cancer may have difficulty swallowing as a temporary side effect of chemotherapy or radiation therapy to the throat or chest area, or because of a treatable infection of the mouth or esophagus, such as thrush, which is a yeast infection.

Trouble swallowing can cause gagging, coughing, or regurgitation of food, weight loss, food build-up in the mouth, drooling, excessive saliva, little or no saliva, pain in the throat or mid-chest when you swallow, and white patches or coating on the inside of the mouth.

How to cope with difficulty swallowing. Here are some eating tips you may want to keep in mind to help you swallow more easily. Use a local anesthetic or pain reliever, such as viscous lidocaine (by doctor's prescription) or liquid Tylenol, if you have pain. Tilt your head

Reducing Pain or Soothing Eating and Swallowing Difficulties

	Sore Mouth or Throat	Mouth Sores	Bleeding in Mouth	Dry Mouth	Difficulty Swallowing
Use prescription topical medications	X				
Rinse often to soothe sore mouth, gums, and tissues.	X		X		
Don't rinse with commercial mouthwash preparations, use dental floss, use lemon or glycerine swabs, or wear loose dentures, which can cause irritation.		X	X		
Have ice chips or frozen juice cubes available to suck on; avoid hard candies if mouth is bleeding.			X		
Apply cream or salve to lips to prevent dryness.			X	X	
Don't use aspirin, which can increase the tendency to bleed; do check labels of all over-the-counter drugs because some contain aspirin.			X		

back and forth to help foods and liquids flow to the back of the throat for swallowing.

Sometimes thicker fluids are more easily tolerated than thin liquids. Don't force yourself to eat if you cannot swallow. Follow your health care team's instructions for any special eating techniques. You may also want to select from the following thickening products:

- ❧ Gelatin: Use to form a soft gel with cakes, cookies, crackers, sandwiches, pureed fruits, and other cold foods. Mix one tablespoon of unflavored gelatin in two cups of liquid until dissolved and pour over food. Allow food to sit until it is saturated.
- ❧ Tapioca, flour, and cornstarch: Use to thicken liquids. Note that these must be cooked before using.
- ❧ Commercial thickeners: Follow label instructions and use to adjust a liquid's thickness.

Coping with Swallowing Problems

Swallowing problems were such a surprise, since they came and went with no identifiable cause. The most important thing I had to remember was to drink and swallow small amounts, slowly...all the time.

—*Kathi*

177

What to Eat When You Have Trouble Swallowing

Your doctor may recommend a liquid diet to help you eat while you're having difficulty swallowing. If thin liquids are recommended for you, try coffee, tea, soft drinks, nutritional drinks, Italian ice, sherbet, broth, and thin cream soups. Once you can eat a pureed thick-liquid diet without swallowing challenges, you may move on to a mechanical thick-liquid diet of more substance that is easy to chew. High-protein drinkable yogurt such as Nouriche is easy to swallow and may help rejuvenate normal bacteria levels.

	Pureed Thick-Liquid Diet:	Mechanical Soft Thick-Liquid Diet
High Protein	Thickened milk, yogurt without fruit, cottage cheese, sour cream, pureed meat, poultry, and fish, casseroles, soft scrambled eggs	Milk, yogurt, cheeses, sour cream, all eggs, ground meats and ground meat casseroles, fish, sandwiches made with ground meats or spreads
Breads, Cereals, Rice, and Pasta	Cooked cereals such as Cream of Wheat and Cream of Rice, slurried (a slurry is a thin paste of water and flour stirred into hot dishes as a thickener. When spread on top of bread or cake, it add moisture and makes dry foods like this easier to swallow.)	Soft breads, graham crackers, cookies, soft cold cereals in milk, pancakes, waffles, pasta, rice
Fruits and Vegetables	Pureed fruit and vegetables without seeds and skins, mashed potatoes	Bananas, canned fruit, soft well-cooked or pureed vegetables
Beverages, Desserts, and Miscellaneous	Thickened juices and nectars, thick milkshakes, thickened broths and cream soups, custard, pudding, slurried cakes and cookies syrups, honey, butter, margarine, spices as tolerated	All beverages, soft desserts that do not require much chewing, such as ice cream, sherbet, flavored gelatin, pudding, custard, soft cakes and cookies, syrups, honey, butter, margarine, spices

©2000 American Dietetic Association; "The Clinical Guide to Oncology Nutrition: Patient Education Materials." Used with permission.

- ❧ Pureed vegetables and instant potatoes: Use in soups. Note that these alter the food's flavor.
- ❧ Baby rice cereal: Use to make a very thick product.

Call the doctor about any of the following symptoms:

- increased gagging, coughing, or choking
- severe sore throat
- red, shiny mouth or ulcers in the mouth or on tongue
- temperature higher than 100.5 degrees F (taken orally)
- difficulty breathing
- chest congestion

Appetite Challenges

Changes in appetite, because of feelings of fullness or changes in taste and smell, for example, can make getting the calories and nutrients you need a challenge. Don't be afraid to break the rules and eat what you want when you want to eat it. Try eating smaller meals and snacks more often. If breakfast foods taste best to you at night or you crave a hearty dinner at lunchtime, feel free to depart from traditional meals.

MANAGING CHANGES IN TASTE AND SMELL

One common oral problem that occurrs after chemotherapy and radiation therapy is an inability to taste normally. Radiation may cause a change in the sweet, sour, bitter, and salt tastes; this usually resolves two to three months after therapy.

Cancer and its treatments can cause changes in your senses of taste and smell. Your favorite foods may not taste great to you anymore. If you are having a problem with food aversions, try foods or beverages that are different from ones you usually eat. To keep from developing food aversions, try new foods and nutritional drinks when you're feeling well. Eat lightly on the morning of or several hours before receiving chemotherapy. Don't taste something new when you smell odors that are distasteful to you. Also, keep your mouth clean by rinsing and brushing, which in turn may improve the taste of foods.

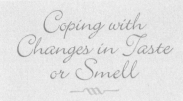

Coping with Changes in Taste or Smell

If the smell of food cooking makes you feel queasy or takes away your appetite, try lighting a scented candle before cooking and leaving it lit throughout the meal. In my case, lighting a vanilla-scented candle was the only way I could even begin to eat.

—*Kathi*

Listen to your body. Even if you've never craved a food before, eat it if your body wants it. If you want tuna, eat it. Your body knows what you need.

—*Elizabeth*

A baked sweet potato or pumpkin pudding is easy to bake and has no odor, which can be helpful for chemo patients sensitive to food smells.

—*Norma Jean*

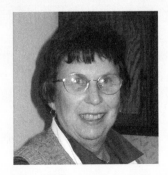

179

How to cope when you can't stand the smell of food. Try the following when food odors make you feel ill:

- ❧ Ask another person to cook for you. Ask them to take off any food covers to release food odors before entering your room or eating area.
- ❧ Rely on prepared foods from the deli.
- ❧ Avoid eating in a room that has cooking odors or other smells. Cook outside on the grill or use boiling bags to reduce cooking odors. Kitchen fans and small portable fans can be used to direct food odors away from you.
- ❧ Don't fry or cook foods with a strong odor like onions, cruciferous vegetables, heavy meats, or fish.
- ❧ Get creative; if smells from cooking appliances make you queasy, consider placing the coffeemaker or toaster oven in the far end of the house or the garage.
- ❧ Order take-out food to avoid preparing food (and creating strong smells) at home.
- ❧ Prepare cold food such as a sandwich, pasta salad, and cottage cheese or yogurt instead of hot food, because odors are in the rising steam.

How to cope when food just doesn't taste the same. Chemotherapy, radiation therapy, or cancer itself can make food taste funny. You may taste a bitter or a metallic taste or not taste much of anything. You may turn your nose up at sweet foods or at meat and poultry. Try these ways of coping as your tastes evolve:

- ❧ Try using plastic utensils if you have a metallic taste while eating.
- ❧ Serve foods cold or at room temperature. This can decrease the foods' tastes and smells, making them easier to tolerate.
- ❧ Rinse your mouth with tea, ginger ale, salted water, or water with baking soda before eating to help clear your taste buds.
- ❧ Season foods with tart flavors such as lemon wedges, lemonade, citrus fruits, vinegar, and pickled foods. (If you have a sore mouth or throat, do not use this tip.)

Coping with Changes in Taste or Smell

I found that sucking on ice chips between every couple of bites of food helped numb my taste buds and allowed me to eat more.

—Bertha (Birdie)

If your favorite food doesn't taste right—or leaves you completely cold, stay away from that food until you are better. That way you will have one more positive thing to look forward to in your recovery. My first "correct" taste of tortillas with cheese and salsa was yet another opportunity for celebration! I also completely lost my sweet tooth during treatment. The first time a big chewy brownie tasted good to me was an absolute joy.

—Kathi

- Increase the sugar in foods to increase their pleasant tastes and decrease salty, bitter, or acidic tastes.
- Flavor foods with onion, garlic, chili powder, basil, oregano, rosemary, tarragon, barbecue sauce, mustard, ketchup, or mint.
- Suck on lemon drops or mints or chew gum to get rid of an unpleasant taste in your mouth after eating. (If you have diarrhea, avoid sugarless candies and gums.)
- Freeze and eat foods such as cantaloupe, grapes, oranges, and watermelon.
- Get a dental checkup to rule out dental problems that could be causing a bad taste in the mouth.
- Clean your mouth and teeth regularly.

What to eat when food doesn't taste or smell like it used to. Rather than force yourself to eat foods that taste bad to you, find substitutes for those foods. If red meat doesn't taste right, stick with other protein sources, including chicken, turkey, fish, eggs, cottage cheese, cheese, yogurt, or tofu. Consider the following tips and options as well:

- Try eating eggs for protein; they may still be appealing if meat is not.
- Eat fresh vegetables, as they may be more appealing than canned or frozen ones.
- No-salt-added or low-salt canned soups or vegetables may have a metallic taste. You may want to avoid them unless you have high blood pressure and have been advised to eat a low-salt diet.
- You may be able to eat mild pasta dishes and milk products.
- Fruit smoothies and frozen desserts like sorbet or sherbet may be appealing.
- Carrot peel often tastes extremely bitter to people having cancer treatment. Peeled, sweet baby carrots or peeled large carrots won't have this bitter flavor.

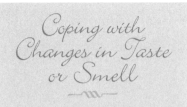

Coping with Changes in Taste or Smell

During treatment, my sense of smell was magnified immensely and my sense of taste, greatly diminished. The smell of food cooking virtually eliminated any appetite I may have had, and some odors prompted immediate vomiting. By accident I discovered that if I sat by a burning vanilla candle during a meal, I was able to reduce my nausea and consume larger portions. Burning vanilla candles during cooking was also helpful. (Other candle scents did not work the same way for me, and overly strong, sweet scents worsened my nausea and sometimes induced vomiting.)

—Kathi

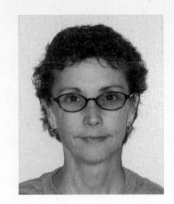

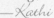

181

A person with a poor or no appetite eats much less than they normally would, or does not eat at all. Loss of appetite or poor appetite is one of the most common problems that occur with cancer and its treatment. Sometimes loss of appetite is a result of side effects of treatment, such as nausea, vomiting, difficulty swallowing, feeling full, or changes in food's taste or smell that make a person feel like not eating. Tumor growth, depression, or pain can also make you uninterested in food. Speak to your health care team about how best to address these causes of poor appetite.

Many people find that their appetite is greatest in the morning. Take advantage of this and eat more then. Consider having your main meal of the day early, and have liquid meal replacements later on if you don't feel so interested in eating.

How to cope with appetite challenges. Most people lose their appetite for just a day or two; for others, it's an ongoing concern.

Ways to cope with treatment side effects:

- Eat food cold or at room temperature to decrease its smell and taste.
- Drink beverages between meals instead of with meals, since drinking liquids at mealtime can lead to early fullness.
- Ask your doctor about medications to help relieve constipation, nausea, pain, or other side effects you have.

How to eat when you have appetite challenges. Whatever the reason for your loss in appetite, the following suggestions may help you cope:

- Eat often enough:
  - Keep snacks within easy reach so you can have something easy to eat whenever you feel like it. Cheese and crackers, muffins, peanut butter, and fruit are good possibilities.
  - Take portable snacks such as peanut butter crackers or small boxes of raisins with you when you go out.

Coping with Loss of Appetite

Very often the servings at restaurants are huge and would be too much to eat even if I weren't ill. When my meal is brought to me, I request a "doggie box" and leave half (or less—only as much as my stomach is capable of handling) of the meal on my plate. Looking at less food seems more manageable and actually convinces my mind that I can eat. The added advantage is that I already have my next meal prepared!

—Susan

Ask for restaurants' lunch menus so you can order smaller portions. Large servings can be overwhelming.

—Norma Jean

Caregivers, don't obsess over your loved one's inability to enjoy what were once favorite foods or beloved meals—they will enjoy them again.

—Charles S.

- Eat as much as you want, but try to eat at least a little bit of food.
- Start the day with breakfast. Eat at mealtimes rather than waiting to get hungry.
- Eat small, frequent meals of favorite foods. It may be easier to eat more that way, and you won't get so full.

❧ Build up your appetite and motivate yourself to eat:
- Make eating more enjoyable by eating with friends, setting the table with pretty dishes and flowers, or playing your favorite music or watching a television show.
- Think of food as a necessary part of treatment.
- Try light exercise an hour before meals.
- If okay with your doctor, try having a glass of beer or wine before eating.

❧ Increase calories and protein:
- Try liquid or powdered meal replacements such as "instant breakfast" when it is hard for you to eat food.
- Try to keep easy-to-eat foods that are high in calories on hand, such as pudding, gelatin, ice cream, yogurt, and milkshakes. (See the High-Calorie, High-Protein Shake and Drink Recipes in the *Recipe Resource Section* of this book for inspiration.)
- Avoid eating low-calorie foods that fill you up, such as lettuce, broth, and diet soft drinks.
- Keep high-calorie, high-protein snacks on hand, such as hard-cooked eggs, luncheon meats, peanut butter, cheese, granola bars, and nutritional supplements.

Eating well and eating enough are important to your recovery from treatment. But don't force yourself to eat; you may make yourself ill. Instead, try to increase your appetite and your motivation to eat, and make sure to eat high-calorie, high-protein foods when you feel interested in eating.

Coping with Loss of Appetite

Caregivers, be patient with loved ones with cancer, as eating can be a problem, especially during chemo. Don't push food if your loved one isn't eating. Offer soft foods like soup or yogurt.

— Melissa

My Reach to Recovery visitor gave me this tip: During chemotherapy treatment, eating small meals more frequently is often easier than facing three traditional-sized meals each day.

— Sally

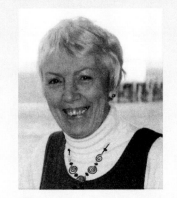

If You Can't Eat Enough

If treatment side effects make it too difficult for you to have even liquid supplements or many small meals a day, you do have other options to get the nutrients you need.

With tube feeding (also called enteral nutrition), a small, thin, flexible tube is placed into the nose and threaded into the stomach to provide liquid nutrients when a person cannot eat enough. The tube can also be placed surgically into the stomach (gastrostomy) or intestine (jejunostomy).

Tube feeding can be an effective way to nourish your body. The idea of being fed through a tube can be off-putting, but many people use this efficient method of "eating" when other methods don't work out for them.

Liquid formulas provide the nutrients you need and eliminate the pressure of mealtimes or eating food you find it difficult to face. With tube feeding, you can eat what appeals to you or not eat at all. You can eat when it suits you—when you're relaxing, watching television, or reading at home.

On those days when you can't eat at all, don't worry. Do what you can to make yourself feel better. Come back to eating as soon as you can, and let your doctor know if this problem doesn't get better within a couple of days.

How Should I Eat after Treatment Is Over?

Chapter 13

Eating Well Every Day

MORE AND MORE PEOPLE WITH CANCER live long, healthy lives after treatment. Living a healthy lifestyle after treatment includes both balanced dietary choices and physically active habits. Eating well during treatment is important, but eating well—and including physical activity —are also important as you recover from treatment and look toward a future beyond cancer.

Healthful Eating after Treatment

You've been conscious of the role of eating well in your overall health throughout treatment; now you may wonder how nutritional and exercise factors can affect your risk of cancer recurrence (cancer that comes back after treatment, whether in the same place as the original cancer, in the lymph nodes, or after spreading to another area of the body) or the development of another cancer, late effects of cancer treatment, and your quality of life.

Although we know a lot about how nutrition and physical activity influence the incidence of cancer, we know less about how they affect cancer recurrence. Most research has focused on which foods prevent cancer in the first place.

Even though the scientific evidence for advice on nutrition and physical activity after cancer is much less certain than for cancer prevention, the American Cancer Society recommends following the standard cancer prevention nutrition

After Cancer, People Often Adopt Healthy Lifestyles

Many people make positive changes in their lives after a cancer diagnosis: eating healthier meals, exercising, and taking vitamins.

This shift to controlling a person's own health is a positive, important step—not only during cancer treatment, but after treatment ends. Two-thirds of those interviewed in one study made at least one change in their behavior after a diagnosis of cancer. Approximately 40 percent improved their diet; 20 percent became physically active; and others began taking multivitamins. Those interviewed reported that their efforts improved their quality of life.

Another study showed that many women made positive dietary changes in the year after they were diagnosed with breast cancer, typically following nutritional guidelines recommended for overall health and cancer prevention. The women who made changes in their diet were concerned about recurrence, coping with and establishing a sense of control over cancer, and improving their prognoses.

More study is needed into the effects of dietary and lifestyle changes on cancer recurrence and new cancers; meanwhile living according to the cancer prevention guidelines outlined in this book will benefit your overall health.

and physical activity guidelines to prevent a second cancer or cancer recurrence. These guidelines stress a diet rich in vegetables and fruits (at least five servings a day) and low in saturated fat, particularly fats from animal sources. Being physically active on a regular basis and drinking alcohol only in moderation also are important. These simple, daily dietary and physical activity choices can fortify the body's defenses and may be especially helpful to people after cancer treatment, when their bodies are recovering and may need an extra boost. Make sure to also work with your medical team to develop a follow-up care plan and follow guidelines for increased cancer screening.

Because people who have been diagnosed with cancer may also be at risk for other cancers, heart disease, diabetes, and osteoporosis, the guidelines established to prevent these diseases are especially important for people who have had cancer. The amounts of fats, protein, and carbohydrates recommended for prevention are also appropriate for people who have had cancer.

Food, Supplements, and Diets after Treatment

If cancer and its treatment have weakened your body, your health care team may recommend that you continue taking a daily multivitamin/mineral supplement after treatment. But research on the role of other foods, supplements, and dietary regimens in the health of people who have had cancer is in its infancy. By some estimates, more than 80 percent of people use dietary supplements or special diets to maintain their health after treatment, despite a lack of scientific evidence of their effects.

Although many commercial supplements claim to boost the immune system, some can actually inhibit the immune system. Be wary of taking high supplemental doses of any nutrient or making dramatic dietary changes—a deficiency of any essential vitamin or mineral during treatment recovery can also weaken the immune system. For more information about vitamins, minerals, and supplements, see chapter 5.

Rely on the knowledge you've gained about these factors as related to your health during treatment—except for interactions with treatment, you can expect much the same results from them now that you're finished as you could during treatment. You're likely eager to preserve your health, so do your research before relying on potentially powerful foods, supplements, and diets sometimes targeted at people who have had cancer, such as herbals, supplements, and soy. (For more information about these topics, see chapters 3 and 5.)

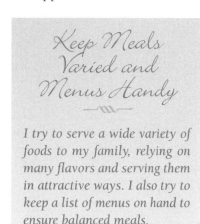

Keep Meals Varied and Menus Handy

I try to serve a wide variety of foods to my family, relying on many flavors and serving them in attractive ways. I also try to keep a list of menus on hand to ensure balanced meals.

—*Annette*

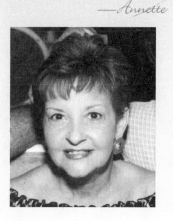

A New Eating Plan: Healthful Eating for Life

Once treatment is over, your ideal nutrition and wellness plan will rebuild muscle strength and help correct problems like anemia or problems with organ functions. Eating enough and being physically active are crucial for a speedy recovery. Your dietitian and other members of your health care team can set up a plan tailored to your needs.

A diet rich in a variety of vegetables, fruits, whole grains, and legumes (beans) reduces cancer risk in people who have never had cancer. These foods

189

Studying Nutrition and Recurrence

Several large-scale, long-term studies are evaluating the effects of various dietary factors on cancer recurrence or secondary cancers. Here is a look at some promising studies that are currently underway:

The Women's Healthy Eating and Living (WHEL) Study

Researchers for the Women's Healthy Eating and Living (WHEL) study are studying women between the ages of 18 and 70 who have been diagnosed and treated with stages I, II, or IIIA breast cancer to find out if a low-fat, plant-based diet might prevent cancer recurrence.

Study leaders hope to determine how the many nutrients in vegetables and fruits that can prevent cancer will affect the health of people relying on them as a main component of their diet after treatment. By considering women's overall diets, those running the study report hope to learn more about the way combinations of food can affect the recurrence of cancers. Study results won't be available until 2006, but when they become available, they may resolve many questions about the effect of diet on risk of cancer recurrence.

The Women's Intervention Nutrition Study (WINS)

The Women's Intervention Nutrition Study (WINS) is testing whether a low-fat diet (where fat makes up only 15 percent of total calories), along with drug therapy, will reduce breast cancer recurrence and improve survival in women with localized breast cancer (an early stage of breast cancer that's confined to one area).

Researchers are studying whether women who eat a low-fat diet has higher rates of survival without cancer than those that didn't change eating habits. They will also compare the two groups' rates of breast cancer recurrence. They expect to determine whether or not the group on the low-fat diet show higher rates of cancer-free survival and lower rates of recurrence.

Nurses' Health Study

This 27-year-old study—phases I and II—looks at women's use of hormones, diet, and lifestyle factors to determine their effects on health. Researchers primarily use questionnaires to assess these lifestyle factors. These ongoing studies are among the largest investigations for major chronic diseases in women and have resulted in many research findings about women and their health.

In recent years, researchers have become interested in the increasing number of people in this study who have had cancer. They have published one preliminary study which indicated that women with breast cancer who ate a diet rich in poultry, fish, and vegetables lived longer than those who didn't. Researchers in this study continue to investigate lifestyle factors which may help women with cancer live longer and healthier lives.

contain vitamins, minerals, and phytochemicals that help the body fight cancer. This diet may also significantly reduce the risk of cancer recurrence and secondary cancers.

Eating well will help you regain your strength, rebuild tissue, and feel better overall. And making positive changes to your diet will help you feel empowered in the process of staying well and feeling good.

EASE INTO HEALTHFUL COOKING AND EATING

Even if your treatment is over and you're feeling much better, you still may not feel completely like your old self. You may not become very interested in eating right away. After all, side effects may have challenged you for some time, and your appetite and desire to enjoy food may have waned along the way. Some of the foods you turned to for nutrition during treatment may not appeal to you as much now. Fighting cancer may have made you tired and you may not be interested in cooking or planning meals right away.

Refer to the food safety information in chapter 10 if you need a refresher on how to keep your kitchen and food free of bacteria and safe to eat. Here are some other ways to help you ease into eating well and cooking without overdoing it.

Take it easy. Don't get overly ambitious; enjoy a simple dinner at home when you first get back into cooking and eating.

- Think about ways you used to make mealtime special and try them again, whether it's candlelight and cloth napkins, a picnic in front of the TV, or having a friend over to share a leisurely lunch.
- Don't be afraid to ask a friend or family member for help with cooking or shopping. Your support system is still important while you're recovering from cancer treatment.
- Take advantage of the supermarket's washed and cut produce, seasoned meat or fish, and prepared foods to make mealtimes easier.

Shop for health. Here are some easy ways to bring healthy choices into the house.

- Buy a new fruit, vegetable, or whole-grain product each time you shop for groceries.
- Choose low-fat milk and dairy products.
- Go easy on saturated fat, salt, sugar, alcohol, and smoked or pickled foods.
- Choose small portions (no more than six to seven ounces a day) of lean meat and poultry without skin.

Good Grilling

Although cooking meats at high temperatures creates carcinogens, chemicals that may increase the risk of cancer, you can still enjoy grilling. Remember the following tips:

- Choose lean cuts of meat and trim excess fat from meat.
- Line the grill with foil and poke small holes in the foil so some fat can drain down but not all the smoke can come back onto the meat.
- Avoid charring meat and don't eat any part that is especially burned and black.
- Marinate meats with a vinegar- or lemon juice-based marinade and a little oil before grilling to prevent the formation of carcinogens.
- Pre-cook meat a bit inside the house then drain away the juices before putting the meat on the grill.
- Watch portion size; aim for a three-ounce meat portion (about the size of a bar of soap). (You might want to start by halving your usual portion if this is a drastic change in portion size. Consider supplementing with grilled vegetables—see below.)
- Grill marinated vegetables, veggie burgers, or veggie hot dogs. Plant-based foods don't form cancer-promoting substances when cooked on the grill.

Now you're cooking. Cut corners on time and effort while making family favorites.

- Make familiar, easy-to-prepare recipes.
- Try out some new "quick and easy" dishes with your favorite flavors in them.
- Cook enough for two or three meals and freeze portions for later. (This works especially well with casseroles and many soups.)
- Decrease the amount of calories in your meals by baking or broiling foods.
- If you are overweight, reduce the amount of calories in your diet and increase your activity. Choose activities that you enjoy.

Get your "five a day." Rethinking your food ratios is an easy way to make healthy choices. Fill your plate with two-thirds vegetables, fruits, whole grains and beans and one-third (or less) meat and dairy products. Some simple ways to increase your intake of plant-based foods:

- Try hearty meatless meals a couple of times a week, like spinach lasagna or vegetarian chili.

- Test out plant-based foods that can substitute for meat, like tofu, tempeh, and beans, or try mushrooms and eggplant for a firm, meat-like texture. All of these foods will fill you up, too. Some easy choices are marinated, roasted portabello mushrooms, baked eggplant with tomatoes and onion, or firm tofu mixed into stir fry or a salad.
- Experiment with one new produce item each time you grocery shop—try making a mango salsa by adding some onion, cilantro, and red bell pepper; add some julienned jicama to your salad; or bake a spaghetti squash and serve as a side dish.
- Choose 100 percent juice and whole-wheat breads at breakfast. Add raisins, dried cranberries, or apple slices to your oatmeal, and add berries or other fruit to your cereal.
- Snack on bell pepper strips, baby carrots, or an orange.

Each fruit and vegetable contains its own special combination of vitamins, minerals, and antioxidants. Buy a variety of produce so your body gets a shot at lots of different foods.

Watch the weight. Cancer treatments may have caused you to gain or lose weight. Talk to your doctor about your ideal healthy weight and how to achieve it after treatment.

Your doctor, nurse, or dietitian should be able to offer strategies for gaining weight that will work for you post-treatment. They may suggest more frequent meals that incorporate high-protein snacks, liquid nutritional products, home-made milkshakes, peanut butter, hummus and vegetables, whole-grain bread and reduced-fat cheese. These foods can help you increase your weight slowly.

Talk to your doctor if you gained weight during treatment and would like to return to your normal weight. Attempts to lose extra pounds should be slow and careful and should only happen after you have recovered from treatment. (One exception may be women with breast cancer, who may benefit from slow, healthy weight loss during treatment and follow a weight loss plan developed by their health care team.) Rely on vegetables, fruits, and other plant-based foods that are high in nutrients and low in calories and saturated fat.

One third of cancer deaths are related to diet and inactivity. About 186,000 lives a year could be saved if people changed those lifestyle habits. Obesity will soon surpass smoking as the leading cause of preventable deaths, and many of those deaths will be from cancer. But people don't realize how much risk there

Calculate Your Body Mass Index (BMI)

The body mass index (BMI) is a ratio of weight to height that is a commonly used indicator of a person's amount of body fat. The BMI can be used as a general measure to help you gauge whether your weight is healthy, although the BMI may not be accurate for people with very low or very high levels of muscle mass. Before taking any steps to change your weight, consult your health care team.

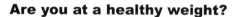

Are you at a healthy weight?

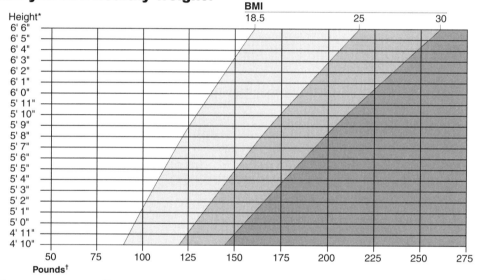

☐ **Healthy Weight**   ◻ **Overweight**   ◼ **Obesity**   * Without shoes. † Without clothes.

The BMI (weight-for-height) ranges shown above for adults. They are not exact ranges of healthy and unhealthy weights. However, they show that health risk increases at higher levels of overweight and obesity. Even within the healthy BMI range, weight gains carry health risks for adults.

Directions: Find your weight on the bottom of the graph. Go straight up from that point until you come to the line that matches your height. Then look to find your weight group.

➢ BMI of 25 defines the upper boundary of healthy weight
➢ BMI of higher than 25 to 30 defines overweight
➢ BMI of higher than 30 defines obesity

Table reprinted from *The Report of the Dietary Guidelines Advisory Committee on the Dietary Giudelines for Americans, 2000*, United States Department of Agriculture.

Will Healthier Snacks Catch On?

The surgeon general notes that obesity has reached epidemic proportions in the U.S. Large snack companies are beginning to develop new, healthier products in the hope of reaching customers' waistlines and wallets. Dietitians and others in the health care industry have clamored for healthier options, citing snack foods' role in people's unhealthy eating habits. Efforts to cut unhealthy sugars, refined carbohydrates, and unhealthy fat, add ingredients such as vegetables, remove some unhealthy oils, and bake instead of fry snack food would all add up to healthier snacking options.

Some fast food companies have responded to the calls for action by broadening their menus to include healthier options like salad and yogurt, and removing some unhealthy oils from French fries, for example. Trans fatty acids in the oils used to make many snacks and fast foods raise blood cholesterol. The Food and Drug Administration (FDA) will require manufacturers to list trans fat content on food and dietary supplement Nutrition Facts panels by 2006.

is in being overweight. A 2002 survey reported that only one percent of participants realized that avoiding being overweight could also help them avoid a higher risk of cancer.

Obesity may increase the risk of breast cancer recurrence by altering the metabolism of estrogen and other hormones.

Trim the saturated fat. Cutting down on saturated fat will help your overall health and help prevent heart disease. But we do need to eat some fat to keep our bodies running smoothly. Olive oil, canola oil, nuts, and fish like salmon, halibut, and cod are sources of "good" fats.

The WINS and WHEL studies (see the *Studying Nutrition and Recurrence* section on page 190 of this chapter for more information) are looking into the effects of low-fat dietary patterns on breast cancer recurrence and survival. Because of a lack of evidence, no dietary recommendations can be made about extremely low-fat diets for preventing a cancer recurrence. The Institute of Medicine recommends that "good" fats make up 20 to 35 percent of your diet. Talk to your doctor or dietitian and make sure your diet remains balanced and that you get the nutrients and calories you need to maintain a healthy body weight.

Eat out wisely. Eating fewer calories and understanding simple ways to control your portions will help you eat out without pigging out. As you explore these ideas for eating delicious restaurant foods without blowing your diet, remember these two especially important tips:

- If you are going to eat out, think about what you are eating the rest of the day so you can plan well and not blow your "calorie budget."
- Restaurants are in the business of serving customers. Don't be afraid to ask for items specially prepared the way you want them.

When you know you're going to eat out, think about what foods you'll choose over the whole day. For example, plan on a light lunch if you'll eat out at dinnertime. Try not to skip meals, which may make you overindulge later. And most importantly, try not to show up at the restaurant famished. If you'd like to splurge on a higher calorie entrée, plan to skip dessert, and commit to sticking to your plan once in the restaurant.

Eating out doesn't have to wreak havoc with your diet. Try some of the following tactics to help make restaurant foods fit into your own eating plan:

- Get exactly what you want by ordering each item separately (a la carte). For example, one chicken enchilada easy-on-the-sauce, side salad, and fruit dessert instead of the #8 enchilada plate with rice, refried beans, sour cream, and guacamole.
- Ask how dishes are prepared and request that the cook grill the chicken, steam the vegetables, bring sauces and salad dressings on the side, or put just a dollop of cream sauce on the pasta primavera and add extra grilled vegetables.
- Don't tempt yourself! Have the waiter remove the bowl of chips or peanuts or the basket of bread after you've had a small portion. Calories from mindless nibbling can add up before you know it.
- Limit alcohol. It's high in calories, has few nutrients, and can weaken your willpower.

The following foods and methods of preparation are likely your best choices to help you stay within your healthy eating plan:

- clear broth-based soups like Chinese wonton or hot and sour soup, consommé, tortilla soup, or minestrone
- raw vegetables (crudités) with a small amount of low-calorie dip

- lettuce or spinach salads with vegetables and dressing on the side (go easy on the bacon bits, croutons, cheese, and mayonnaise-based items like macaroni salad or tuna salad—¼ cup tuna salad = 190 calories)
- steamed vegetables with a slice of lemon; grilled veggies if not drenched in oil
- meats that are grilled (but not charred), broiled, roasted or baked without added fat (choose seafood that is broiled, baked, steamed, blackened, or poached—think tender sole poached in parchment with broth, savory vegetables and herbs)
- a reasonable portion of steak—three to six ounces; other lean meat cuts served au jus, with a piquant fruit sauce, or stir-fried with vegetables (go easy on the rich sauces)
- a baked potato with a pat of butter or small amount of sour cream (top with broccoli, lean chili, or salsa)
- sandwiches on whole wheat, pita, multigrain breads; with lean deli meats and cheeses; mustard, relish, ketchup, or light mayonnaise (add flavor and vitamins with roasted sweet peppers, lettuce, tomato, jalapenos, and a small amount of chopped olives)
- fresh fruit, sherbet, and angel food cake are good choices for dessert

It Doesn't Hurt to Ask

When eating out, you can always request that your food be prepared healthier by asking for no salt, less oil, or no sauce (especially cream-based, high-fat sauces), for example. Order grilled instead of fried, when possible. Most chefs are happy to comply with your special healthy requests.

—*Mardi*

Look for the following descriptions to uncover higher calorie menu choices: pan-fried, sautéed, battered, breaded, au gratin, cheesy, creamy, buttered, deep-fried, béarnaise, or crispy—as in the "crispy," deep-fried tortilla bowl holding the salad.

Portion police. Eating smaller portions of food is one of the easiest ways to cut back on calories—but it can also be one of the most challenging, with the current trend of super-sizing. Huge portions, all-you-can-eat buffets, and extra-large "single servings" of chips, candy bars, and other snack foods can all contribute to overeating.

Even bagels have become super-sized, which gives this reasonably healthy breakfast item a high calorie count. Bakeries and grocery stores often carry jumbo bagels that measure four and a quarter inches across and contain 300–400 calories each. A regular, three-inch-diameter bagel has about 150 calories and counts as two servings of bread in the grain group.

What a Normal Portion Looks Like

How do you know a reasonable portion of food when you see it? It may be smaller than you think. Try to visualize the objects mentioned below when eating out, planning a meal, or grabbing a snack. For example, the amount of meat recommended as part of a healthy meal is three to four ounces—and it will look to be the same size as a deck of cards. According to one study, the typical portion size of food items on the market is at least twice as large as the U.S. Department of Agriculture standard for portions, sometimes eight times as large. Aiming to lower your portion sizes is a positive step even if you don't lower them to the portion goals below. Supplementing with other healthy choices may help satisfy your stomach.

- one ounce meat: size of a matchbox
- three ounces meat: size of a deck of cards or bar of soap—the recommended portion for a meal
- eight ounces meat: size of a thin paperback book
- three ounces fish: size of a checkbook
- one ounce cheese: size of four dice
- medium potato: size of a computer mouse
- two tablespoons peanut butter: size of a ping pong ball
- one cup pasta: size of a tennis ball
- average bagel: size of a hockey puck.

To eat smaller portions try the following ideas:

- When eating out:
  - Order regular portion sizes instead of jumbo sizes. Choose a regular hamburger at your favorite fast food stop instead of the larger burger and save about 150 calories. Have the small fries instead of the super-sized and save about 300 calories. Order the small soda. It has about 150 fewer calories than the large one. (Diet sodas have few or no calories.)
  - Try an appetizer, half an entrée, or share a meal with a friend and order an extra side salad.
  - Ask for half the entrée to be wrapped up to go before the food is brought to the table. Eat it for lunch the next day.

❧ At home:
- Don't "eat from the bag." When snacking, place a few chips, crackers or cookies in a bowl to help prevent overeating.
- Buy single portions of snack foods so you're not tempted by the whole bag or box.
- Like butter and sour cream on your baked potato? Mayonnaise and cheese on your sandwich? Cream cheese on your bagel? Use half the amount you usually do.

Special Concerns

You may have coped with treatment side effects for some time. Now that your treatment has ended, so will most of the eating-related effects of treatment. Sometimes side effects like poor appetite, dry mouth, change in taste or smell, difficulty swallowing, or significant weight loss may persist. If this happens to you, talk to your health care team so you can work together on a plan to address any remaining problem.

ONGOING EATING CONCERNS

Some people are in treatment for a long time. Others may have had surgery to remove part of their stomach or intestines, or radiation to the abdomen that affects their eating and digestion. If you have ongoing eating-related concerns, ask your doctor and dietitian for more information about how to cope with specific long-term issues. They can help developing a plan that meets your dietary needs.

LIVING WITH ADVANCED CANCER

Although many individuals are cured or monitor cancer as a controllable chronic disease, others may live with advanced cancer for many years. Nutrition can be an important part of creating and maintaining a sense of well-being. Eating well may improve quality of life for people with advanced cancer. If you have advanced cancer, rely on foods that are easy to tolerate.

Although many people with advanced cancer lose weight, adapting food choices and eating patterns can help prevent weight loss, meet nutritional needs, and manage symptoms and side effects like pain, constipation, and loss of appetite. Medications can help minimize symptoms like pain or constipation that may interfere with eating. Being physically active as you are able may help to increase appetite and also relieve constipation. Other medications (such as megestrol acetate) may help increase your appetite. Nonsteroidal anti-inflammatory drugs may help stabilize your nutritional status, and some evidence indicates that omega-3 supplements may stabilize or improve your nutritional status, body weight, and functioning. Other types of nutritional support can help if you cannot eat enough. Talk to your health care team about preventing malnutrition and weight loss.

Some level of physical activity is probably positive for people with advanced cancer, since physical activity—even if you are confined to bed—may help increase appetite, reduce constipation, and counteract fatigue. But there is very limited research on exercise in people with advanced disease. Therefore, talk to your health care team about recommendations for nutrition and physical activity and your individual needs and situation.

See the *If You Can't Eat Enough* section on page 184 of chapter 12 for information about nutrition options for people with special concerns.

Staying Active

A growing number of studies have examined exercise during recovery and long-term survival after cancer treatment, mainly studying women with breast cancer or people who have received bone marrow transplants. Overall, exercise has shown important benefits in physical fitness and overall quality of life. No studies have examined the effects of exercise on cancer recurrence or overall survival after cancer treatment, but several current studies will provide data on this issue in the next few years.

In the meantime, other studies suggest that exercise is related to the prevention of some cancers and other chronic diseases like heart disease and diabetes, and it is likely that these preventative benefits will also be found to apply to people who have had cancer. Physical activity is therefore probably helpful in preventing second cancers and other chronic diseases. For the general population, the ACS and other health organizations recommend at least 30 minutes of moderate physical activity at least five days per week. These levels of activity have not been studied or tested specifically in people who have had cancer, but the health benefits of exercise are in general greater the greater the intensity of physical activity and time spent exercising. (Excessive over-training can result in an increased risk for a lowered immune system, however.)

After treatment for any cancer, increasing body strength and recovering your pre-treatment fitness level (or improving it) is important. The benefits of exercise in improving overall quality of life are well known. In studies, increasing physical activity has positively influenced heart rate, lung capacity, and lean body mass in people who have had cancer (these effects are similar to those in people who have not had cancer). If you have had or continue to have physical limitations or have not been physically active in the past, plan a physical activity plan with your health care team before jumping into an exercise regimen.

Exercise can help you regain strength and flexibility, relieve stress, and help you maintain an optimal weight. Physical activity prods your body to produce new red blood cells and may also strengthen the immune system. Regular exercise can also reintroduce a sense of autonomy that you may feel you have lost during treatment.

A well-rounded exercise program includes aerobic exercise (which increases the heart rate and the amount of oxygen your body uses), strength training using weights, and flexibility exercises. Even when performed regularly in small increments, this balanced approach to physical activity provides real benefits for the body.

Performing moderately intense aerobic exercise frequently—three to five times per week for a total of 30 to 60 minutes each day—is a good goal. This exercise can be accomplished in ten-minute increments throughout the day. Walking, running, cycling, swimming, and stair climbing are examples of activities that exercise the major muscle groups. Vigorous housework and yard work count, too—as does any activity that makes you breathe as intensely as you do when walking quickly.

A well-rounded program of resistance or strength training will help improve muscular strength and endurance, body composition, and flexibility. General stretching exercises involving the major muscle and tendon groups can help maintain range-of-motion in joints and overall flexibility as adults age.

Many Americans feel they simply don't have the time to increase their physical activity. However, much like healthful eating, increasing physical activity can be achieved by making a few simple changes in your routine. Here are some helpful ways to be more aerobically active:

- Use stairs rather than an elevator.
- If you can, walk or bike to your destination.
- Exercise at lunch with your workmates, family, or friends.
- Take a ten-minute exercise break at work to stretch or take a quick walk.
- Walk to visit co-workers instead of sending an email.

- Go dancing with your spouse or friends.
- Plan active vacations rather than only driving trips.
- Wear a pedometer every day and watch your daily steps increase. (Aim for and try to work up to 10,000 per day—walking instead of driving to a nearby friend's house, parking far from the store and walking through the parking lot, and strolling through the neighborhood help the steps add up.)
- Join a sports team.
- Use a stationary bicycle while watching TV.
- Plan your exercise routine to gradually increase the days per week and minutes per session.

If you are able, engage in at least moderate aerobic activity for 30 minutes or more on five or more days of the week.

You may be fatigued and unable to be physically active for long just after you finish treatment. Consult your doctor before beginning an exercise program or increasing your physical activity, and ask for advice on creating an individualized exercise program. Then start slowly and working up to a moderate level of exercise as you are able. Incorporating exercise as a permanent lifestyle change is the ultimate goal.

Physical Activity and the Elderly

For those over age 65, a balanced exercise program can help restore joint and muscle flexibility. By including flexibility training—such as stretching exercises—in their exercise programs, elderly adults can offset naturally occurring muscle and skeletal changes that significantly impair daily life. Flexibility exercises can improve range of motion and function of joints, and can also be important in preventing musculoskeletal injuries. (In addition, exercise helps relieve depression in the elderly and helps keep elderly minds sharp.)

Those over age 65 may need longer periods of time to adapt to an exercise program, but healthy elderly people and elderly individuals with health challenges can make significant increases in strength and muscle mass through resistance and strength training. Older people can be up and moving seven days a week and should also spend time on five of those days doing extra flexibility exercises or walking. Start with five minutes of stretching, then add a few minutes of walking. Build up as you can.

Special Concerns with Physical Activity after Treatment

If you are confined to bed because of cancer, treatment, or other reasons, talk to your health care team about physical therapy to help you stay strong and keep your joints moving. If you've been in bed a long time, your endurance, your muscle strength, and your fitness level have decreased. This can make everyday tasks more tiring. Those who are limited to bed can cope with fatigue, stress, and emotional lows with light physical activity.

If you've been dehydrated and have had an imbalance of electrolytes, your activity level may be low. Make sure to drink plenty of liquids with even limited activity. If you've had cancer in your bones or treatment that affected your bone strength, abrupt jumping or vigorous twisting might fracture the bone; talk to your health care team about appropriate activities. If you have lymphedema following surgery or radiation to the lymph nodes under the arm for breast cancer, you'll want to use your affected arm for everyday activities four to six weeks after treatment, but be careful not to overdo activity. Talk to your health care team about tennis or weightlifting, which could tire out your arm.

Community and gym programs often offer options for people beginning physical activity for the first time or taking it up after a time of inactivity. Classes may focus on people with special physical activity needs. If you were extremely active before treatment, take it slow when you first get back into exercise. Your health care team and an exercise specialist can help you develop activities appropriate for your post-treatment health and can reevaluate if you grow stronger.

The effects of physical activity on heart disease and diabetes have not been studied in people with cancer, but there is no reason to believe that outcomes would be different from those in the general population. Resistance exercise (resistance training and weight lifting) has been reported to improve bone strength in persons without cancer, but the effectiveness of resistance exercise programs on osteoporosis in people with cancer is not yet known.

Women who go through menopause during or after treatment and men who are treated with long-term anti-androgenic medications are at high risk for osteoporosis. Studies of segments of the general population at risk for osteoporosis indicates that people at risk for osteoporosis after treatment might benefit from resistance training for its potential bone strengthening effects. Improved lean body mass and balance from physical activity might also reduce the risk of falls and fractures. Clinical trials are underway testing the effects of aerobic and resistance exercise on bone density in women who have had post-menopausal breast cancer.

People with lymphedema may also find health benefits in exercise—specifically range of motion exercises—if their surgeons have cleared them for physical activity. The benefits and risks of resistance training in people with lymphedema have not been extensively studied, but some studies suggest that despite some concerns that physical activity might negatively affect lymphedema, resistance training does not increase the risk for lymphedema or worsen lymphedema.

Other situations to make note of and discuss with your health care team as you consider a plan for physical activity:

- If you have severe anemia, wait to exercise until you have recovered from treatment.
- If you have compromised immune function, avoid public gyms and other public places until your white blood cell counts are back to normal. Exercise at home or outdoors for a time instead. (If you have had a bone marrow transplant, your health care team may advise you to avoid exposure to public places with risk of microbial contamination, such as gyms, for a year after your transplant.)
- If you have severe fatigue from therapy, you may not feel up to an exercise program. Instead, your health care team might encourage you to do ten minutes of stretching exercises each day.
- If you have significant neuropathies (tingling and burning sensations or weakness or numbness in your hands and feet), you may not be able to exercise your affected limbs. You may also feel off balance and may prefer a reclining bicycle, for example, than walking on a treadmill or outdoors.

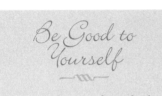

Be Good to Yourself

We're in charge of our bodies, so we need to take care of them. Eat good, fresh fruit and veggies, drink lots of good water, take vitamins, cut out junk food and sodas, and cut down on red meat. Keeping a positive attitude and having faith helps, too.

—*Gloria*

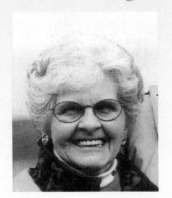

Treatment may be a challenging time for people with cancer. After treatment, many people are ready to live life to its fullest—and are willing to take extra steps to make sure they're around to enjoy more of it. Making simple changes in your daily life like eating for health, being active, and keeping a healthy weight can help you reach those goals.

Easy Meals to Rely on during and after Treatment

Simple, Healthy Recipes for the Whole Family

EARLIER IN THIS BOOK you read about tips for shopping and stocking the pantry to save time and hassle when you're concentrating on treatment. You also read about the types of foods you may want to eat or avoid during different cancer treatments to help prevent or alleviate side effects.

This chapter contains specific recipes and meal ideas for people with cancer and their families as well as for friends who want to help. These nutritious, tasty meals can be made with minimal effort. Many people with cancer and caregivers have provided their own favorite recipes for this section, allowing us to offer you their wisdom and the delicious recipes that can help provide important nutrients before, during, and after treatment. Their recipes are introduced with personal notes.

Recipes for Healthful Eating

Feel free to adapt recipes to fit your current eating and digestion status—for example, if a recipe contains small amounts of dairy products and you are lactose intolerant, feel free to substitute non-dairy items or omit them. Add the dairy products later if you're better able to digest them. Omit onions or tomatoes if they bother a sore mouth, and replace with milder vegetables that are still packed with flavor such as mushrooms, squash, or peppers. If you're trying to add calories to your diet, disregard directions for "low-calorie" or "light" versions of dairy products and use the full-calorie options. Unless you have diarrhea, include more whole grains by substituting whole-wheat pastas wherever pasta is called for in these recipes.

The legend that accompanies each recipe indicates which treatment side effects it may help alleviate and which it may aggravate. You may want to use these legends to help you eat to cope with eating- and digestion-related effects of treatment. Each person's reaction to treatment is different, and everyone may not be affected the same way by dish ingredients, so you may need to experiment to see which foods make you feel better or worse. Meanwhile, let this legend guide you during treatment if you're experiencing constipation, diarrhea, a sore throat or mouth, a dry mouth or difficulty swallowing, or lactose intolerance, for example.

Some side effects—such as fatigue, nausea and vomiting, decreased appetite, and dehydration—don't easily translate into dish-by-dish recommendations. To help alleviate fatigue, focus on dishes high in calories and protein. Nausea and vomiting can be brought on by different foods in different people; mild, bland foods and clear liquids are safer bets than strong spices, fatty or fried foods, or spicy flavors. If you have a decreased appetite, try eating multiple small meals a day, and try to eat concentrated protein and calories so that what you do eat packs a nutrient punch. If you're trying to stay hydrated, focus on dishes with high liquid contents and explore the many beverage options presented here.

After finishing treatment for your cancer, a balanced diet rich in vegetables, fruits, and whole grains, with red meat only in moderation may reduce the risk of recurrence or other cancers, as well as other chronic diseases such as heart disease, diabetes, and hypertension. (See chapter 13 for more information about nutrition after cancer treatment.)

Recipe analyses were provided by the University of Arizona Cancer Center, Nutrition and Behavior Measurement Unit. Nutrient amounts have been rounded to the nearest tenth of a number. When a range of servings is provided (Makes 2–4 servings), nutrient amounts listed correspond to the higher number of servings.

Sample Menus

These dish combinations are tasty anytime, including when the whole family is eating together, both before and after treatment; they may also be used if you're coping with side effects during treatment. Mix and match the recipes here to create delicious meals.

Many of the beverage options here are especially nutritious if you add high-calorie, high-protein powders to them. After treatment, they're still wonderful as breakfasts, desserts, or snacks. They can also serve as meals on their own if your appetite is decreased or if it's difficult to eat.

DEALING WITH CONSTIPATION

If you're constipated, make sure to take in plenty of liquids throughout the day.

Menu 1:
Peanut Butter Snack Spread
Turkey Vegetable Soup
Blueberry Peach Crisp

Menu 2:
Fruity Drink
Orzo Salad
Black Bean Cakes

COMBATING DIARRHEA

Menu 1:
Dilled Carrots
Lemon-Spiked Chicken
Baked Apples

Menu 2:
Zucchini Bites
Linguini with Tomato, Basil, and Capers
Pumpkin Custard

MINIMIZING DRY MOUTH OR DIFFICULTY SWALLOWING

Menu 1:
Tuscan White Bean Salad
Cheesy Vegetable Soup
Peach Yogurt Frost

Menu 2:
Potato Soup
Rosemary Beef with Shallot Sauce
Chocolate Cocoa Drink

COPING WITH LACTOSE INTOLERANCE

Menu 1:
Eggplant Dip
Hearty Vegetable Barley Soup
Fruit Smoothie

Menu 2:
Gazpacho
Green Bean, Wild Rice, and
Veggie Burger Casserole
Lactose-Free Double Chocolate Pudding

Fruity Drink

This drink offers lots of nutrients and much-needed liquids. The fresh juice means you'll have none of the preservatives or refined sugars that are in many store-bought juices.

—*Karen*

Note: Keep frozen berries on hand to make this drink—you can purchase them without preservatives or added sugar.

May be appropriate for:
Constipation
Dry Mouth or Difficulty Swallowing
Lactose Intolerance

May not be appropriate for:
Diarrhea
Sore Mouth

Half of an orange or tangerine
3 slices of pineapple
1 apple
6 large strawberries

Half of a banana
12 green or red grapes
½ cup raspberries
½ cup blackberries

Juice all ingredients in a juicer.

Makes 2–4 servings.

Calories: 114; Protein: 1.3 g; Fat: 0.9 g; Cholesterol: 0 mg; Dietary fiber: 6 g

Veggie Drink

This yummy recipe will help energize you. It contains many nutrients to help you be good to your body.

—*Karen*

Note: Red or yellow peppers will enhance the sweetness of the dish. Feel free to exclude the cabbage, broccoli, and green pepper if you're not able to digest them without difficulty. If you have gastrointestinal challenges, you may want to instead include beets, carrots, celery, and fresh ginger, fresh lime juice (unless you have mouth sores), and serve cold.

May be appropriate for:
Constipation
Dry Mouth or Difficulty Swallowing
Lactose Intolerance

May not be appropriate for:
Diarrhea

1 beet
4 carrots
3 broccoli florets with stems
Handful of parsley

¼ head of cabbage
½ green pepper
2 stalks celery
Handful of spinach

Juice all ingredients in a juicer.

Makes 2–4 servings.

Calories: 59; Protein: 2.4 g; Fat: 0.4 g; Cholesterol: 0 mg; Dietary fiber: 4.4 g

Note: For the following recipes,
follow these basic instructions unless otherwise directed:

Place all ingredients in a blender container or prepare in large container with a hand-held blender. Cover and blend on high speed until well blended. Chill before serving. Store unused drinks in refrigerator or freezer. Add 1 to 2 tablespoons of powdered milk to each recipe to increase protein content.

If you cannot tolerate milk or milk products,
ask your health care professional for appropriate recipe ideas.

Sherbet Shake

This refreshing shake is a cinch to make and offers lots of calories and protein too.

Note: If you're lactose intolerant, substitute lactose-free milk
and sorbet for the milk and sherbet in this recipe.

1 cup sherbet
½ cup whole milk
½ teaspoon vanilla extract

Makes 1 serving.

Calories: 285; Protein: 5.6 g; Fat: 7 g; Cholesterol: 25.5 mg; Dietary fiber: 0.7 g

May be appropriate for:
Diarrhea
Dry Mouth or Difficulty Swallowing
Lactose Intolerance
Sore Mouth or Throat

May not be appropriate for:
Constipation

Cottage Cheese Smoothie

This thick, protein-packed drink has some tang to it
because of the cottage cheese.

⅓ cup cottage cheese
½ cup vanilla ice cream
¼ cup prepared fruit-flavored gelatin

Makes 1 serving.

Calories: 245; Protein: 11.9 g; Fat: 10.4 g; Cholesterol: 39.5 mg; Dietary fiber: 0 g

May be appropriate for:
Diarrhea
Dry Mouth or Difficulty Swallowing
Sore Mouth or Throat

May not be appropriate for:
Constipation
Lactose Intolerance

Classic Instant Breakfast Milkshake

This protein-packed favorite provides nutrients in a concentrated form.
For variety, add strawberries, blueberries, peaches, or any other
fresh or frozen fruit.

May be appropriate for:
Diarrhea
Dry Mouth or Difficulty Swallowing
Sore Mouth or Throat

May not be appropriate for:
Constipation
Lactose Intolerance

½ cup whole milk
1 envelope Instant Breakfast mix (such as Carnation)
1 cup vanilla ice cream (add flavorings and
   different ice creams for variety)

Makes 1 serving.

Calories: 463; Protein: 12.6 g; Fat: 18.7 g; Cholesterol: 76.8 mg; Dietary fiber: 0.5 g

Peach Yogurt Frost

This frosty, tangy drink is great as dessert or as a high-calorie snack.
Replace ice cubes with frozen fruit for a twist.

May be appropriate for:
Diarrhea
Dry Mouth or Difficulty Swallowing
Sore Mouth or Throat

May not be appropriate for:
Constipation
Lactose Intolerance

1 envelope vanilla instant breakfast mix
1 cup whole milk
½ cup peach yogurt
6 to 10 crushed ice cubes

Makes 1 serving.

Calories: 398; Protein: 17.4 g; Fat: 9.6 g; Cholesterol: 40.4 mg; Dietary fiber: 0.9 g

Chocolate Cocoa Drink

This cool, creamy chocolate drink is easy to make too.

May be appropriate for:
Dry Mouth or Difficulty Swallowing
Sore Mouth or Throat

May not be appropriate for:
Constipation
Diarrhea
Lactose Intolerance

1¼ cups vanilla ice cream
½ cup whole milk
1 package hot chocolate mix
2 teaspoons sugar

Makes 1 serving.

Calories: 538; Protein: 10.7 g; Fat: 23.1 g; Cholesterol: 89.2 mg; Dietary fiber: 1.6 g

Banana Milkshake

This dessert-like shake is also high in potassium.
Using frozen bananas will help thicken the drink.

1 whole ripe banana, sliced
Vanilla extract (a few drops)
1 cup milk

Makes 1 serving.

Calories: 262; Protein: 9.2 g; Fat: 8.7 g; Cholesterol: 33.2 mg; Dietary fiber: 2.8 g

Recipe courtesy of the National Cancer Institute,
Eating Hints for Cancer Patients: Before, During, and After Treatment.

May be appropriate for:
Dry Mouth or Difficulty Swallowing
Sore Mouth or Throat

May not be appropriate for:
Constipation
Diarrhea
Lactose Intolerance

Fruit Smoothie

It's fine to use frozen or fresh fruits in this smoothie, or a mix of both.

—*Karen*

*Note: Other delicious fruit combinations include pears and peaches, pineapple
and mango with coconut extract and orange juice, and apricots and raspberries. Feel
free to substitute pomegranate juice, such as Pom Wonderful, for the orange juice.*

½ cup blueberries
½ cup strawberries
½ cup blackberries
½ cup raspberries
1½ cups orange juice
Soy or protein powder

Makes 2–4 servings.

Calories: 114; Protein: 6 g; Fat: 0.9 g; Cholesterol: 0 mg; Dietary fiber: 5 g

May be appropriate for:
Constipation
Dry Mouth or Difficulty Swallowing
Lactose Intolerance

May not be appropriate for:
Diarrhea
Sore Mouth or Throat

I devised the three following high-protein, high-calorie drinks when my husband could not stand any of the canned liquid supplements and lost a lot of weight with his end-stage lymphoma. They can be valuable for people who experience weight loss.

—*Eleanor*

High-Protein Milk

Note: Using 1 quart powdered milk in 1 quart whole milk—which has 3½ percent milk fat—slightly reduces calories and protein.

**May be
appropriate for:**
Dry Mouth or
Difficulty Swallowing
Sore Mouth or Throat

**May not be
appropriate for:**
Constipation
Diarrhea
Lactose Intolerance

Mix together:
1 package instant milk powder (such as Milkman)
1 quart extra-rich milk (milk that contains 4 percent milk fat or more)

Makes 4 1-cup servings.

Calories: 185; Protein: 9.9 g; Fat: 10 g; Cholesterol: 40.9 mg; Dietary fiber: 0 g

Hot Drink

**May be
appropriate for:**
Dry Mouth or
Difficulty Swallowing
Sore Mouth or Throat

**May not be
appropriate for:**
Constipation
Diarrhea
Lactose Intolerance

Heat in microwave or on stove:
1 cup (8 ounces) High-Protein Milk (recipe above)

Add and heat:
1 package Instant Breakfast, any flavor (such as Carnation)
4–6 heaping teaspoons Ovaltine

Makes 1 serving.

Calories: 346; Protein: 14.4 g; Fat: 10.4 g; Cholesterol: 43.2 mg; Dietary fiber: 0.9 g

Flavor can be varied by substituting chocolate Carnation Instant Breakfast, chocolate-flavored Ovaltine, and chocolate ice cream. Omitting the peanut butter changes the caloric and protein content. (Do not substitute diet Instant Breakfast!)

— Eleanor

Milkshake

Note: Natural peanut butter generally contains peanuts and peanut oil, without the preservatives and hydrogenated oils in other peanut butters. (When hydrogenated oils are made, trans fats are produced that contribute to artery-clogging deposits.)

Mix in blender:
1 cup (8 ounces) High Protein Milk (see recipe on page 214)
¼ cup egg substitute (such as Second Nature brand)
1 envelope vanilla Instant Breakfast (such as Carnation)
½ cup vanilla ice cream
1 tablespoon creamy peanut butter
3 tablespoons malted milk powder (such as Carnation)

Makes 1 serving.

Calories: 648; Protein: 27.8 g; Fat: 27.3 g; Cholesterol: 76.2 mg; Dietary fiber: 2.1 g

May be appropriate for:
Dry Mouth or
Difficulty Swallowing
Sore Mouth or Throat

May not be appropriate for:
Constipation
Diarrhea
Lactose Intolerance

Eggplant Dip

I like to keep a lot of al dente vegetables in the refrigerator
for dipping into this yummy, nutritious dip.

— Verna

Note: Red bell peppers may be easier to digest than green bell peppers.

1 eggplant	1 small green or red bell pepper, minced
¾ teaspoon salt	¼ cup olive oil (add more as needed)
¼ teaspoon pepper	2 tablespoons vinegar or lemon juice
1 small onion, minced	

Bake whole eggplant in oven at 375 degrees F until very tender, about 45 minutes. Let cool. Scoop eggplant pulp into a bowl and mash. Add vegetables and seasonings. Chill and serve in a small bowl surrounded by whole-grain bread, vegetables, or crackers.

Makes 4–6 servings.

Calories: 113; Protein: 1 g; Fat: 9.3 g; Cholesterol: 0 mg; Dietary fiber: 2.7 g

*May be
appropriate for:*
Constipation
Dry Mouth or
Difficulty Swallowing
Lactose Intolerance

*May not be
appropriate for:*
Diarrhea
Sore Mouth or Throat

Apple/Prune Sauce

*Note: Feel free to use unsweetened applesauce
or add a squeeze of lemon to balance the sweetness.*

⅓ cup unprocessed bran
⅓ cup applesauce
⅓ cup mashed stewed prunes

Blend all ingredients and store in refrigerator.
Take 1–2 tablespoons of this mixture before bedtime, then drink 8 ounces of water. (Make sure you drink the water, or this mixture will not work to relieve constipation.)

Makes 16 servings.

Calories: 13; Protein: 0.3 g; Fat: 0.1 g; Cholesterol: 0 mg; Dietary fiber: 0.9 g

*Recipe courtesy of the National Cancer Institute,
Eating Hints for Cancer Patients: Before, During, and After Treatment.*

*May be
appropriate for:*
Constipation
Dry Mouth or
Difficulty Swallowing
Lactose Intolerance

*May not be
appropriate for:*
Diarrhea

Zucchini Bites

These baked treats are a great, easy start to a meal.

Note: Peel the zucchini if you're experiencing diarrhea. Use regular baking mix if you're trying to add calories to your diet. If the smell of Parmesan cheese makes you feel nauseous, replace with a less pungent-smelling cheese or omit.

2 medium zucchini, cut into ¾-inch rounds
½ cup reduced-fat baking mix (such as Bisquick)
2 tablespoons grated Parmesan cheese
Olive oil cooking spray
½ teaspoon garlic salt
½ teaspoon paprika

Preheat oven to 350 degrees F. Spray both sides of zucchini slices with cooking spray. Coat with baking mix. Place zucchini slices in skillet or on cookie sheet and sprinkle with garlic salt, paprika, and Parmesan cheese. Bake for 15 minutes or until slightly browned. Serve immediately.

Makes 8 servings.

Calories: 43; Protein: 1.9 g; Fat: 1.1 g; Cholesterol: 1.2 mg; Dietary fiber: 0.8 g

Adapted from the American Cancer Society's *Celebrate! Healthy Entertaining for Any Occasion.*

May be appropriate for:
Constipation
Diarrhea

May not be appropriate for:
Dry Mouth or Difficulty Swallowing
Lactose Intolerance
Sore Mouth or Throat

Hummus

Tahini is a high-fat paste made from sesame seeds. Eating hummus with whole-wheat pita and baby carrots or broccoli is a quick way to get calories and protein.

¼ cup tahini
1 teaspoon cumin (or more, to taste)
½ teaspoon salt
2 large cloves garlic, finely chopped
3 tablespoons lemon juice
3 tablespoons hot water
1 19-ounce can garbanzo beans, drained
Chopped fresh parsley

Combine tahini, cumin, salt, and garlic in a small bowl. While mixing, slowly pour in lemon juice, then hot water. Puree garbanzo beans in a food processor. Add tahini mixture and process again. Season to taste. Sprinkle with chopped parsley.

Makes 6–8 servings.

Calories: 158; Protein: 7.4 g; Fat: 5.9 g; Cholesterol: 0 mg; Dietary fiber: 5.9 g

Reprinted from *The American Cancer Society's Healthy Eating Cookbook, Second Edition.*

May be appropriate for:
Constipation
Dry Mouth or Difficulty Swallowing
Lactose Intolerance

May not be appropriate for:
Diarrhea
Sore Mouth or Throat

217

Peanut Butter Snack Spread

This snack provides protein and calories in a yummy form.
Add cinnamon for flavor if you wish.

Note: Natural peanut butter generally contains peanuts and peanut oil without the preservatives and hydrogenated oils in other peanut butters. (When hydrogenated oils are made, trans fats are produced that contribute to artery-clogging deposits.)

1 tablespoon nonfat instant dry milk
1 teaspoon water
1 teaspoon vanilla extract
1 tablespoon honey
5 tablespoons peanut butter

May be appropriate for:
Constipation

May not be appropriate for:
Diarrhea
Dry Mouth or Difficulty Swallowing
Lactose Intolerance
Sore Mouth or Throat

Combine dry milk, water, and vanilla, stirring to moisten. Add honey and peanut butter, stirring slowly until liquid blends with peanut butter. Spread on crackers.

Mixture also can be formed into balls, chilled, and eaten as candy. It keeps well in the refrigerator but is difficult to spread when cold.

Makes 2 6-tablespoon servings.

Calories: 285; Protein: 11 g; Fat: 20.6 g; Cholesterol: 0.4 mg; Dietary fiber: 2.4 g

Recipe courtesy of the National Cancer Institute,
Eating Hints for Cancer Patients: Before, During, and After Treatment.

Easy Minestrone

As I was battling the worst of my nausea and vomiting, a friend called and asked if she could pop by and drop off some soup that she had made. Marilyn's minestrone was the first food I was able to keep down. I loved the taste, and it freezes well. She uses egg pastini, such as Ronzoni, as the pasta.

—*Kathi*

Note: If you want to add tomatoes and their lycopenes to this dish, substitute canned crushed tomatoes and their liquid for half of the beef broth.

1 pound lean ground beef or turkey
1 cup chopped celery (about 4 stalks)
2 carrots, cut into strips or grated (about 16–18 baby carrots)
½ cup chopped onion (about 1 small onion)
2 quarts (5 cans) beef broth
½ teaspoon basil
½ teaspoon oregano
¼ teaspoon pepper
1 cup (6 ounces) small pasta like orzo or pastini
1 10-ounce package frozen, chopped spinach
1 can (20 ounces) chickpeas (optional)
1–2 tablespoons grated Parmesan cheese per serving (optional)

Brown beef in heavy 6-quart pan over medium heat, stirring frequently. Drain fat.

Add celery, carrots, and onion. Cook and stir about 10 minutes or until vegetables are tender. Add broth and seasonings. Cook and simmer 30 minutes. Stir in pasta and spinach. Stir occasionally and cook about 10 minutes or until pasta is tender. Add chickpeas, if desired. Heat thoroughly. Season to taste and serve with grated Parmesan cheese, if desired.

Makes 6–8 servings.

Calories: 412; Protein: 32.3 g; Fat: 11 g; Cholesterol: 44.5 mg; Dietary fiber: 7.9 g

May be appropriate for:
Constipation
Dry Mouth or Difficulty Swallowing
Lactose Intolerance

May not be appropriate for:
Diarrhea

219

Hearty Vegetable Barley Soup

This is a great way to get your vegetables and comfort food at the same time.

—Margaret

Note: Substituting beef broth for some of the water and the beef boullion will help cut the salt.

1 pound lean beef, cut into cubes
1 tablespoon olive oil
Half of an onion, chopped
1 clove garlic, minced
7 cups water
16 ounces canned, diced tomatoes

½ cup barley
½ cup celery, chopped
½ cup carrots, chopped
4 beef boullion cubes
½ teaspoon dried basil
1 bay leaf

Brown meat in oil. Add onion and garlic. Cook until soft and drain. Stir in remaining ingredients and cover. Bring to a boil. Reduce heat and simmer for 50 minutes.

Makes 4–6 servings.

Calories: 255; Protein: 18.6 g; Fat: 11.4 g; Cholesterol: 47 mg; Dietary fiber: 4.1 g

May be appropriate for:
Constipation
Dry Mouth or
Difficulty Swallowing
Lactose Intolerance

May not be appropriate for:
Diarrhea

Cheesy Vegetable Soup

This is an easy way to get your veggies. I use Velveeta, which means plenty of calories to prevent weight loss, too.

—Carol

Note: You may want to substitute vegetables that aren't likely to make you gassy, such as string beans and peas.

6 cups chicken broth
1 14½-ounce can crushed seasoned tomatoes
1 pound broccoli, chopped
½ pound cauliflower, chopped

1 cup carrots, chopped
6 ounces cheddar or part-
   skim mozzarella cheese
Salt and pepper to taste

Heat broth and tomatoes. Add vegetables and simmer until tender. Add cheese and salt and pepper to taste.

Makes 4–6 servings.

Calories: 206; Protein: 15.8 g; Fat: 11.2 g; Cholesterol: 29.7 mg; Dietary fiber: 4.6 g

May be appropriate for:
Dry Mouth or
Difficulty Swallowing

May not be appropriate for:
Constipation
Diarrhea
Lactose Intolerance

Winter Soup

This cozy soup is simple to make and tasty, too. Serve in soup bowls with croutons, cornbread, crackers, or a sprinkle of Parmesan cheese.

2 tablespoons canola or olive oil
1 medium onion, chopped
2 14½-ounce cans fat-free chicken
  broth, either homemade or canned
¾ cup tomato sauce

½ cup macaroni, uncooked
Pepper to taste
1 15-ounce can white beans
  (cannellini or Great Northern
  beans), drained

Heat oil in a large soup pot over medium low heat. Add onion and cook for 3 minutes. Add broth and tomato sauce, bring to a boil, then stir in macaroni. Reduce heat, cover and simmer for 10 minutes. Add pepper to taste, then stir in white beans. Heat mixture thoroughly.

Makes 4–6 servings.

Calories: 219; Protein: 11.7 g; Fat: 5.8 g; Cholesterol: 0 mg; Dietary fiber: 5.7 g

Reprinted from *The American Cancer Society's Healthy Eating Cookbook, Second Edition.*

May be appropriate for:
Constipation
Dry Mouth or Difficulty Swallowing
Lactose Intolerance

May not be appropriate for:
Diarrhea

Turkey Vegetable Soup

The lean turkey and many vegetables in this soup make it a lowfat way to get your "five a day."

1 teaspoon canola or olive oil
1 pound lean ground turkey
1 cup onion, diced
1 large clove garlic, minced
2 cups water
1½ cups potatoes, peeled and diced

½ cup carrots, peeled and chopped
2 15-ounce cans tomatoes
1 10-ounce package frozen mixed vegetables
1 teaspoon chili powder
½ teaspoon oregano
½ teaspoon marjoram

In a large pot over low heat, sauté the turkey, onion, and garlic in oil. Drain fat. Add water and potatoes and bring to a boil. Cook 10 minutes. Add carrots and tomatoes and cook 10 minutes more. Add mixed vegetables and spices, cover, and simmer for 15 minutes.

Makes 8 1½-cup servings.

Calories: 153; Protein: 15 g; Fat: 4.1 g; Cholesterol: 37.9 mg; Dietary fiber: 3.4 g

May be appropriate for:
Constipation
Dry Mouth or Difficulty Swallowing
Lactose Intolerance

May not be appropriate for:
Diarrhea
Sore Mouth or Throat

221

Gazpacho

This is a springtime and summertime soup with a little kick—adjust the onion, hot sauce, and garlic powder to your taste. To mix it up a little, substitute tomatoes for the tomato soup and water, and sprinkle with chopped cilantro.

2 cans tomato soup
2 cans water
1 tablespoon olive oil
1 teaspoon salt
Dash hot sauce
Dash garlic powder

1 small onion, chopped
1 cucumber, peeled, seeded, and chopped
1 green pepper, seeded and chopped
1 large can or 2 fresh tomatoes,
    peeled, seeded, and chopped

Mix together first 6 ingredients (tomato soup through garlic powder), then add remaining ingredients. Or blend in the blender or food processor to make a pureed soup.

Makes 8 1-cup servings.

Calories: 66; Protein: 1.3 g; Fat: 2.6 g; Cholesterol: 0 mg; Dietary fiber: 1.4 g

Cream of Broccoli Soup

This is a delicious way to eat cruciferous vegetables and enjoy plenty of flavor in a low-fat, creamy soup.

3 cups broccoli florets and peeled
    stems, finely chopped
1½ cups water
1 tablespoon olive oil
½ cup onion, chopped
1 tablespoon all-purpose flour

3 cups 1-percent fat milk
½ teaspoon salt (optional)
½ teaspoon pepper
¼ teaspoon paprika
¼ teaspoon celery seed
⅛ teaspoon cayenne pepper

Combine broccoli and water in a 3-quart saucepan and bring to a boil. Lower heat, cover, and simmer for 10 minutes. Drain, saving liquid. Add oil to a larger saucepan, add onion, and sauté over low heat until soft. Add flour and continue to cook for several seconds, stirring constantly. Stir in reserved liquid and cook until thickened. Add milk, broccoli, salt, black pepper, paprika, celery seed, and cayenne pepper, mixing well. Warm over low heat before serving.

Makes 6 servings.

Calories: 94; Protein: 5.7 g; Fat: 3.8 g; Cholesterol: 4.9 mg; Dietary fiber: 1.7 g

Reprinted from *The American Cancer Society's Healthy Eating Cookbook, Second Edition.*

Potato Soup

To make this soup appropriate for those with diarrhea, omit the onion, which may upset the stomach.

3 medium potatoes, peeled and cubed
2 cups reduced-sodium chicken broth
2 stalks chopped celery
½ small onion, peeled
1 tablespoon butter
1 tablespoon flour
2 cups reduced-fat milk
2 eggs, hard cooked, peeled, and chopped
Salt and pepper to taste

Cook the potatoes in chicken broth with celery and onion until the potatoes are tender. Blend the mixture in a blender or processor. In a heavy saucepan over low heat, melt the butter and stir in flour to make a paste. Slowly add the milk, stirring or whisking continuously until the mixture is thoroughly blended and heated through. Add the pureed potato mixture. Add chopped eggs that have been pushed through a sieve. Mix well and season with salt and pepper as desired. Serve hot or cold. (This soup thickens when chilled and may need to be thinned with additional chicken broth or milk before serving.)

May be appropriate for:
Dry Mouth or Difficulty Swallowing

May not be appropriate for:
Constipation
Diarrhea
Lactose Intolerance

Makes 4 servings.

Calories: 237; Protein: 11.7 g; Fat: 8.7 g; Cholesterol: 122.9 mg; Dietary fiber: 2.3 g

Orzo Salad

This is a personal favorite. I think I made this flavorful salad a million times last summer.

—*Ivy*

Note: For a version lower in fat and calories, decrease the amount of cheese and oil.

16-ounce package orzo
10 ounces baby spinach,
  washed and chopped
½ pound crumbled feta cheese
½ red onion, chopped

¾ cup pine nuts
Chopped fresh basil to taste
Ground pepper to taste
½ cup olive oil
½ cup balsamic vinegar

Cook orzo 8–10 minutes. Rinse with cold water. In a big bowl, mix everything but oil and vinegar. Toss with oil and vinegar before serving.

Makes 4–6 servings.

Calories: 671; Protein: 18.7 g; Fat: 37.5 g; Cholesterol: 33.6 mg; Dietary fiber: 5.9 g

Asian Salad

This is my favorite salad. It's delicious.

—*Joanne*

Note: For variety, consider adding pineapple chunks and sliced almonds.

Dressing:
3 tablespoons olive oil
2 tablespoons balsamic vinegar
2 packets of Splenda or sugar
Salt and pepper to taste
Package of oriental spice mix
  (from Ramen Noodles)

Salad:
⅓ cup green cabbage, shredded
⅓ cup red cabbage, shredded
⅓ cup green onions, chopped
Small can mandarin oranges
Ramen Noodles, crushed

Whisk together oil, vinegar, Splenda or sugar, and salt and pepper. Add spice mix to taste. Mix with salad ingredients.

Makes 1 serving.

Calories: 918; Protein: 11.1 g; Fat: 57.1 g; Cholesterol: 0 mg; Dietary fiber: 9.2 g

Minestrone Salad

This make-ahead dish includes lots of good-for-you ingredients: whole-wheat pasta, broccoli, and plenty of fiber in the beans and other vegetables. It's low in fat, too. Substitute more of the other vegetables for the broccoli if it upsets your stomach.

12 ounces whole-wheat elbow pasta
1 tablespoon fresh lemon juice
1 16-ounce can Great Northern beans, drained and rinsed
1½ cups reduced-fat Italian salad dressing
2 cups fresh broccoli florets
1 cup zucchini, cut into rounds and sliced into strips
1 cup fresh carrots, cut into rounds
½ cup green onions with tops, chopped
½ cup red and/or green bell pepper, seeded and chopped
Lettuce leaves
Tomato slices for garnish

Cook pasta according to package directions, adding lemon juice to water, then drain. Mix pasta with beans and salad dressing in a large bowl and refrigerate overnight. In a saucepan or steamer, steam broccoli until tender-crisp. Immediately place broccoli into a bowl of ice water to stop cooking process, then drain well. Add broccoli, zucchini, carrots, green onions, and bell pepper to pasta mixture and mix gently. Let stand for 2 to 3 hours before serving. Arrange lettuce on salad plates and spoon salad onto lettuce. Garnish with tomato slices.

Makes 8 servings.

Calories: 293; Protein: 12.1 g; Fat: 6.9 g; Cholesterol: 0.6 mg; Dietary fiber: 7.9 g

Reprinted from *The American Cancer Society's Healthy Eating Cookbook, Second Edition.*

May be appropriate for:
Constipation
Dry Mouth or Difficulty Swallowing
Lactose Intolerance

May not be appropriate for:
Diarrhea
Sore Mouth or Throat

Dilled Carrots

This dish can be made with whole baby carrots if regular carrots taste bitter to you during treatment—or if you simply don't want to chop them.

2 pounds carrots, sliced
⅓ cup fresh parsley, chopped
¼ cup vegetable or chicken broth
3 tablespoons white wine vinegar
1 tablespoon olive oil

2 teaspoons granulated sugar
3 tablespoons fresh dill, chopped, or 1 teaspoon dried dillweed
Salt and pepper to taste

May be appropriate for:

Constipation
Diarrhea
Dry Mouth or Difficulty Swallowing
Lactose Intolerance

May not be appropriate for:

Sore Mouth or Throat

In a saucepan over medium heat, steam carrots over a small amount of water until tender. Drain and place carrots in a large bowl. Combine parsley, broth, vinegar, olive oil, sugar, dill, salt, and pepper in a small bowl and mix well. Pour mixture over warm carrots. Marinate in the refrigerator for several hours before serving.

Makes 8 servings.

Calories: 66; Protein: 1.3 g; Fat: 2 g; Cholesterol: 0 mg; Dietary fiber: 3.2 g

Reprinted from the American Cancer Society's *Celebrate! Healthy Entertaining for Any Occasion.*

Succotash Plus

This is a great mix of vegetables, and the lean sausage gives it great flavor and helps prevent weight gain.

—*Kristi*

Note: Fiesta corn is a mix of corn, onions, bell peppers, and sometimes green chiles.

8 ounces lean smoked sausage (such as Healthy Choice)
½ cup chopped onion
1 can lima beans

1 can fiesta corn
1 can diced tomatoes (seasoned with green chiles or garlic and onion)
1 can mixed carrots and green peas

May be appropriate for:

Constipation
Dry Mouth or Difficulty Swallowing
Lactose Intolerance

May not be appropriate for:

Diarrhea
Sore Mouth or Throat

Cook sausage and onion in nonstick skillet, about 5 minutes, until sausage is brown and onion is tender. Drain fat. Add vegetables and undrained tomatoes. Cook uncovered 8 to 10 minutes until liquid is nearly gone.

Makes 6 servings.

Calories: 267; Protein: 11.6 g; Fat: 11.4 g; Cholesterol: 23.1 mg; Dietary fiber: 6.9 g

Couscous with Almonds, Dried Blueberries, and Parmesan Cheese

This is a fast, easy dish based on a whole grain, couscous. You can substitute dried cranberries or chopped dried apricots for the blueberries if you prefer.

2½ cups fat-free chicken broth
2 teaspoons garlic salt
2 cups couscous
2 tablespoons olive oil
½ cup dried blueberries
2 tablespoons slivered almonds
4 tablespoons grated or shredded Parmesan cheese, divided

In a medium saucepan, bring chicken broth and garlic salt to a boil. Add couscous, stir, and remove from heat. Allow to sit for 5 minutes. Mix in olive oil, blueberries, almonds, and 2 tablespoons of Parmesan cheese. Transfer to serving dish and top with remaining 2 tablespoons of cheese.

Makes 8 servings.

Calories: 238; Protein: 8.8 g; Fat: 6 g; Cholesterol: 2.5 mg; Dietary fiber: 2.8 g

Reprinted from the American Cancer Society's *Celebrate! Healthy Entertaining for Any Occasion*.

May be appropriate for:
Constipation

May not be appropriate for:
Diarrhea
Dry Mouth or
Difficulty Swallowing
Lactose Intolerance

Tuscan White Bean Salad

This quick and easy recipe makes an elegant appetizer or a flavorful side dish for meals. Toss the ingredients together about 45 minutes before serving so the salad can chill in the refrigerator for 30 minutes. Serve with soft pita bread or mashed on top of sliced, toasted Italian bread for crostini.

Salad dressing:
2 tablespoons + 1 teaspoon olive oil, divided
1 garlic clove, minced
1 teaspoon dried oregano
¼ cup cider vinegar

Bean salad:
2 16-ounce cans cannellini beans or Great Northern beans, rinsed and drained
1½ cups diced plum tomato
½ cup chopped Vidalia or other sweet onion
½ cup (2 ounces) crumbled feta cheese
⅓ cup chopped fresh parsley
½ teaspoon salt
½ teaspoon ground pepper

May be appropriate for:
Constipation
Dry Mouth or Difficulty Swallowing
Lactose Intolerance

May not be appropriate for:
Diarrhea
Sore Mouth or Throat

To prepare salad dressing:
In a nonstick skillet, heat 1 teaspoon of olive oil over medium-high heat. Add the garlic and oregano; sauté for 30 seconds. Remove from heat and stir in vinegar.

To prepare the salad:
In a large bowl, combine remaining 2 tablespoons olive oil and the bean salad ingredients. Add the dressing to the bean salad; toss lightly. Cover and chill for 30 minutes before serving.

Makes 8 servings.

Calories: 197; Protein: 10.5 g; Fat: 6.4 g; Cholesterol: 8.3 mg; Dietary fiber: 6.3 g

Adapted from the American Cancer Society's *Celebrate! Healthy Entertaining for Any Occasion.*

Green Bean, Wild Rice, and Veggie Burger Casserole

We eat a lot of chicken, fish, and veggie burgers instead of red meat. This is one of our favorite easy, quick, and tasty made-up meals. It takes 22 minutes to prepare and cook. It's tasty and good for you and it fills you up!

—*Karen*

Note: You may want to buy seasoned or flavored veggie burgers, or season plain burgers with your favorite seasoning blend.

2 cups wild rice, cooked
1 large bag frozen green beans
4 veggie burgers

Microwave green beans 17 minutes. Microwave veggie burgers 5 minutes. Dice burgers. Mix ingredients together before serving.

Makes 4–6 servings.

Calories: 138; Protein: 9.8 g; Fat: 2 g; Cholesterol: 0 mg; Dietary fiber: 4.1 g

May be appropriate for:
Constipation
Lactose Intolerance

May not be appropriate for:
Diarrhea
Dry Mouth or
Difficulty Swallowing
Sore Mouth or Throat

Lemon-Spiked Chicken

This microwaved dish is even more simple than the list of directions makes it seem.
The light lemon flavor and rich mushrooms mix to create a wonderful flavor.

6 chicken breast halves, skinned and boned
2 tablespoons plus 1 teaspoon butter, divided
1½ tablespoons all-purpose flour
½ teaspoon dried tarragon
½ teaspoon salt, optional
¼ pound fresh mushrooms, thinly sliced
¼ cup hot water
1 teaspoon instant chicken boullion
½ lemon, thinly sliced
3 cups cooked brown rice

May be appropriate for:
Constipation
Diarrhea
Dry Mouth or
Difficulty Swallowing
Lactose Intolerance

May not be appropriate for:
Sore Mouth or Throat

Cut each chicken breast half into 8- to 10-inch strips. Place 2 tablespoons butter into a 2-quart glass casserole and microwave on high for 1 minute. Add chicken, then sprinkle with flour, tarragon, and salt. Cover and microwave on high for 4 minutes, stirring at 1-minute intervals. Place remaining 1 teaspoon of butter into a 1-quart glass casserole and microwave on high for 1 minute. Add mushrooms, tossing to mix. Microwave on high for 1½ minutes, stirring after 1 minute. Add to chicken. Combine hot water and bouillon in a small bowl and stir until dissolved. Pour mixture over chicken and arrange lemon slices on top. Microwave on high for 5 minutes or until chicken is tender. Serve over rice.

Makes 6 servings.

Calories: 310; Protein: 29.8 g; Fat: 9.4 g; Cholesterol: 85.2 mg; Dietary fiber: 2.2 g

Reprinted from *The American Cancer Society's Healthy Eating Cookbook, Second Edition.*

Black Bean Cakes

This high-fiber, vegetarian dish is flavorful and great for the whole family. Serve with a salad, such as spinach and toasted pine nuts. Omit the hot sauce and onion if you have a sore mouth or throat; consider serving with salsa if you don't.

Cooking spray
½ medium sweet red bell pepper, diced finely
½ medium onion, diced finely
1 large carrot, sliced into thin coins
1 15-ounce can black beans, rinsed and drained well, mashed slightly
1 4-ounce can green chiles, chopped, undrained
½ cup cooked barley
1 tablespoon Parmesan cheese
¼ teaspoon garlic salt
Dash hot sauce, or to taste
½ cup seasoned breadcrumbs
2 eggs, beaten

Lightly spray a medium nonstick skillet with cooking spray. Over medium-high heat, sauté red pepper, onion, and carrot until tender. Set aside. In a large bowl, mix together beans, green chiles, barley, cheese, garlic salt, and hot sauce. Mix in breadcrumbs, sautéed vegetables, and eggs. Form bean mixture into tablespoon-sized balls. Drop onto nonstick skillet that has been lightly sprayed with cooking spray and heated to medium-high heat. Flatten each ball into a cake with a spatula. Cook 1 minute per side or until crispy and brown.

May be appropriate for:
Constipation

May not be appropriate for:
Diarrhea
Lactose Intolerance
Sore Mouth or Throat

Makes 8 servings.

Calories: 180; Protein: 7.9 g; Fat: 6 g; Cholesterol: 47.3 mg; Dietary fiber: 4.9 g

Reprinted from the American Cancer Society's *Celebrate! Healthy Entertaining for Any Occasion.*

Rosemary Beef with Shallot Sauce

Serve this dish over rice if you wish. Tender lean beef with flavorful sauce
is a nice low-fat meat option.

2 pounds lean round steak, thinly sliced and cut into bite-sized pieces
½ teaspoon black pepper
2 teaspoons fresh rosemary, chopped
½ teaspoon garlic salt
2 teaspoons olive oil
4 shallots, finely chopped
1 medium sweet red pepper, chopped
1 pound mushrooms, sliced
½ cup light sour cream
¼ cup light cream cheese
Rosemary sprigs for garnish

*May be
appropriate for:*
Constipation
Dry Mouth or
Difficulty Swallowing

*May not be
appropriate for:*
Diarrhea
Lactose Intolerance
Sore Mouth or Throat

Season steak pieces with pepper, rosemary, and garlic salt. Heat olive oil
in large skillet over medium-high heat. Add shallots and red pepper; sauté
until tender, about 2 minutes. Add steak and sauté 2 to 3 minutes or until
slightly browned. Add mushrooms and cook until tender. Remove from
heat and mix in sour cream and cream cheese. Garnish with fresh rosemary sprigs, if desired.

Makes 8 servings.

Calories: 195; Protein: 25.9 g; Fat: 7.1 g; Cholesterol: 68.7 mg; Dietary fiber: 1.3 g

Reprinted from the American Cancer Society's *Celebrate! Healthy Entertaining for Any Occasion.*

Greek Chicken with Tomatoes, Peppers, Olives, and Feta

If fresh Roma tomatoes aren't available, use canned tomatoes, which will provide a more vivid color and even more lycopenes.

Greek seasoning salt:
2 teaspoons garlic salt
2 teaspoons lemon pepper
2 teaspoons oregano
2 teaspoons dried mint

4 boneless, skinless chicken breast halves, cut into bite-sized pieces
¼ cup flour
8 teaspoons Greek seasoning salt, divided
1 teaspoon olive oil
1 large onion, sliced lengthwise
1 green pepper, cored, seeded, and sliced lengthwise into strips
3 Roma tomatoes, cut into eighths, or 1½ cups canned tomatoes
3 tablespoons Kalamata olives, chopped
3 tablespoons feta cheese, crumbled

Combine ingredients for Greek seasoning salt. Dredge chicken in flour mixed with 4 teaspoons of Greek seasoning. Heat oil in a large skillet over medium heat and add chicken, sautéing for 3 to 4 minutes until cooked through. Remove chicken from pan and set aside. Add onion to skillet and sauté until tender, about 2 minutes. Add bell pepper and cook another 2 minutes. Return chicken to skillet and cook 1 to 2 minutes, sprinkling with remaining Greek seasoning. Mix in tomatoes. Remove from heat, transfer to serving dish, and sprinkle with olives and feta cheese.

Makes 8 servings.

Calories: 111; Protein: 14.5 g; Fat: 3.8 g; Cholesterol: 39.7 mg; Dietary fiber: 1.1 g

Reprinted from the American Cancer Society's *Celebrate! Healthy Entertaining for Any Occasion.*

May be appropriate for:
Constipation

May not be appropriate for:
Diarrhea
Dry Mouth or Difficulty Swallowing
Lactose Intolerance
Sore Mouth or Throat

233

Linguini with Tomato, Basil, and Capers

Immerse the tomatoes in boiling water (blanching them) for a few minutes so you'll be able to remove the skins more easily. Or use canned, crushed Italian tomatoes in place of the tomatoes and spices and add capers, vinegar, salt, and pepper to the linguini.

2 pounds spinach or whole-wheat linguini, uncooked
4 tomatoes, peeled, seeded, and coarsely chopped
1 cup fresh basil, coarsely chopped
3 tablespoons olive oil, divided
⅓ cup onion, finely chopped
½ cup carrot, finely chopped
½ cup celery, finely chopped
3 cloves garlic, crushed
1 3¼-ounce jar capers, drained and rinsed
3 tablespoons vinegar
Salt and pepper to taste

May be appropriate for:
Diarrhea
Lactose Intolerance

May not be appropriate for:
Dry Mouth or
Difficulty Swallowing
Sore Mouth or Throat

In a large pan of boiling water, cook linguini according to package directions. Drain. Meanwhile, mix tomatoes and basil in a bowl. Set aside. Heat 1 tablespoon of oil in a skillet over low heat. Add onion and sauté until translucent, about 2 to 3 minutes. Add carrot, celery, and garlic and sauté for another minute. Add tomato mixture and simmer, uncovered, for 20 minutes. Add capers, vinegar, salt, and pepper. Drizzle remaining olive oil on linguini, tossing to coat. Place linguini onto a large serving platter and top with sauce.

Makes 8 servings.

Calories: 522; Protein: 16.3 g; Fat: 7.5 g; Cholesterol: 0 mg; Dietary fiber: 5.7 g

Reprinted from the American Cancer Society's *Celebrate! Healthy Entertaining for Any Occasion.*

234

Reduced-Fat Banana Pudding

The fat-free pudding and whipped topping cut the fat considerably from traditional banana pudding, which is great if you're trying to prevent weight gain.

— *Sheila*

1 box fat-free, sugar-free vanilla instant pudding
1 can evaporated skim milk

1 container fat-free whipped topping
2–3 sliced bananas
½–¾ box of reduced-fat vanilla wafers

Mix pudding and milk, then beat until thick. Fold in whipped topping. Refrigerate for 5 minutes. In a serving bowl, layer twice as follows: vanilla wafers, bananas, pudding mix. Top with vanilla wafers and refrigerate until ready to eat.

Makes 6–8 servings.

Calories: 189; Protein: 4.6 g; Fat: 2.4 g; Cholesterol: 1.6 mg; Dietary fiber: 1.3 g

May be appropriate for:
Dry Mouth or Difficulty Swallowing
Sore Mouth or Throat

May not be appropriate for:
Constipation
Diarrhea
Lactose Intolerance

Baked Apples

This simple dessert is appropriate for people who are having most eating- or digestion-related side effects from treatment. Feel free to add ⅛ teaspoon lemon rind to the filling if you don't have a sore mouth and to add ½ cup raisins if you aren't experiencing diarrhea. Sprinkle with crumbled ginger snaps if you wish.

4 large apples
¼ cup (packed) brown sugar

½ teaspoon cinnamon
¾ cup water

Preheat oven to 375 degrees F. Wash and core apples without puncturing bottoms (leave ½ inch of core at bottom; you may want to use a melon baller). Peel skin from the top third of the apple. Combine sugar and cinnamon and fill the apples with the mixture. Bring water to a boil. Place apples cavity side up in an 8 × 8 pan and pour boiling water into and around apples. Bake 60 minutes, basting apples with juices from the pan several times. Remove from heat and let stand 10 minutes, continuing to baste. Serve warm or cold.

Makes 4 servings.

Calories: 178; Protein: 0.4 g; Fat: 0.8 g; Cholesterol: 0 mg; Dietary fiber: 5.9 g

May be appropriate for:
Constipation
Diarrhea
Dry Mouth or Difficulty Swallowing
Lactose Intolerance
Sore Mouth or Throat

235

Pumpkin Custard

Note: Replace the milk with lactose-free milk if you're experiencing diarrhea.

4 egg whites
2 eggs
1 15-ounce can pumpkin
⅔ cup brown sugar
1 tablespoon cornstarch
2 12-ounce cans evaporated skim milk

½ tablespoon vanilla extract
1 teaspoon ground cinnamon
¼ teaspoon ground ginger
¼ teaspoon salt (optional)
Ground nutmeg

Preheat oven to 350 degrees F. Whisk egg whites in a bowl. Gently add eggs, pumpkin, brown sugar, and cornstarch, mixing thoroughly. Add evaporated milk gradually, continuing to stir. Add vanilla, cinnamon, ginger, and salt. Whisk to combine thoroughly. Lightly spray a soufflé dish with nonstick cooking spray. Pour the mixture into the soufflé dish. Sprinkle with a little nutmeg. Bake for 50–60 minutes, until set and custard is lightly browned. Transfer to a wire rack to cool.

Makes 6 servings.

Calories: 112; Protein: 6.4 g; Fat: 0.4 g; Cholesterol: 2 mg; Dietary fiber: 1.8 g

May be appropriate for:
Diarrhea
Dry Mouth or Difficulty Swallowing
Sore Mouth or Throat

May not be appropriate for:
Constipation
Lactose Intolerance

Creamy Frozen Fruit Bars

Serve fresh fruit with these easy dessert bars.

1 cup vanilla yogurt
½ cup all-fruit preserves
1 8-ounce package light cream cheese

Line an 8 × 8 square pan with plastic wrap. Blend all ingredients. Spread evenly in pan. Cover and freeze about 2 hours, until firm. Remove mixture from pan using plastic wrap, cut into four squares, and serve.

Makes 4 servings.

Calories: 275; Protein: 8.6 g; Fat: 9.6 g; Cholesterol: 30.7 mg; Dietary fiber: 0.6 g

May be appropriate for:
Dry Mouth or Difficulty Swallowing
Sore Mouth or Throat

May not be appropriate for:
Constipation
Diarrhea
Lactose Intolerance

Lactose-Free Double Chocolate Pudding

If you're lactose intolerant, you can still have your chocolate
and eat it too with this dessert.

2 ounces baking chocolate
1 tablespoon cornstarch
¼ cup granulated sugar

1 cup nondairy creamer,
 soy formula, or lactose-free milk
1 teaspoon vanilla extract

Melt chocolate in small saucepan. Measure cornstarch and sugar into pan.
Add part of the creamer, soy formula, or lactose-free milk and stir until
cornstarch dissolves. Add the remainder of the liquid. Cook over medium
heat until warm. Stir in chocolate until mixture is thick and comes to a
boil. Remove from heat. Blend in vanilla and cool.

Makes 2 servings.

Calories: 282; Protein: 4 g; Fat: 9.8 g; Cholesterol: 0 mg; Dietary fiber: 2.7 g

Recipe courtesy of the National Cancer Institute, *Eating Hints for Cancer Patients: Before, During, and After Treatment.*

*May be
appropriate for:*
Dry Mouth or
Difficulty Swallowing
Lactose Intolerance
Sore Mouth or Throat

*May not be
appropriate for:*
Constipation
Diarrhea

Blueberry Peach Crisp

This quick, delicious dessert contains fresh fruit and whole-grain oats and just
3 tablespoons of butter for 8 servings, so it's relatively healthy, too.

6 cups fresh peaches, peeled and sliced
2 cups fresh blueberries
⅓ cup + ¼ cup light brown sugar,
 divided

2 tablespoons all-purpose flour
1 tablespoon cinnamon, divided
1 cup quick-cooking oats
3 tablespoons butter

Preheat oven to 350 degrees F. In a 2-quart baking dish, combine peaches and
blueberries. Combine ⅓ cup brown sugar, flour, and 2 teaspoons cinnamon in
a small bowl and mix well. Add to peaches and blueberries, tossing to mix.
Combine oats, ¼ cup brown sugar, and 1 teaspoon cinnamon in a bowl. With
a pastry blender or fork, cut in butter until crumbly, then sprinkle over fruit.
Bake for 25 minutes or until fruit is just tender and mixture is bubbly.

Makes 8 servings.

Calories: 222; Protein: 3 g; Fat: 5.3 g; Cholesterol: 11.7 mg; Dietary fiber: 5.1 g

Reprinted from the American Cancer Society's *Celebrate! Healthy Entertaining for Any Occasion.*

*May be
appropriate for:*
Constipation
Lactose Intolerance

*May not be
appropriate for:*
Diarrhea
Dry Mouth or
Difficulty Swallowing
Sore Mouth or Throat

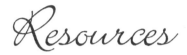

Resources

American Cancer Society

The American Cancer Society (ACS) is the nationwide community-based volunteer health organization dedicated to eliminating cancer as a major health problem by preventing cancer, saving lives, and diminishing suffering from cancer, through research, education, advocacy, and service. For more information about cancer, educational materials, patient programs, and services within your community, contact us:

Toll-free: 800-ACS-2345 (800-227-2345)

Web site: *http://www.cancer.org*

About the Resources

Listings in this section represent organizations that operate on a national level and provide some type of service or resource to consumers related to cancer, cancer research, or public health. This list is designed to offer a starting point for seeking information, support, and needed resources. Most of the organizations listed here can be contacted via phone, fax, or e-mail, and some through a Web site. Many of the Web sites provide much of the same information that is available by postal mail. Some organizations are solely Web-based and will require Internet access. Keep in mind that new Web sites appear daily while old ones expand, move, or disappear entirely. Some of the Web sites or content outlined below may change. Often, a simple Internet search will point to the new Web site for a given organization. The American Cancer Society Web site provides links to outside sources of cancer information as well (*http://www.cancer.org*; search for Related Web Sites).

There is a vast amount of information on the Internet. This information can be quite valuable to the general public in making decisions about their health. However, since any group or individual can publish on the Internet, it is important to consider the credentials and reputation of the organization providing information. Internet information should not be a substitute for medical advice.

The American Cancer Society does not necessarily endorse the agencies, organizations, corporations, and publications represented in this resource guide. This guide is provided for assistance in obtaining information only.

Organizations Providing Health and Cancer Information

Agency for Healthcare Research and Quality (AHRQ)
Office of Health Care Information,
Executive Office Center
2101 East Jefferson Street, Suite 501
Rockville, MD 20852
Phone: 301-594-1360
Web site: *http://www.ahrq.gov*

The AHRQ, an office within the U.S. Department of Health and Human Services (HHS; see page 244), provides consumers with science-based, easily understandable information that will help them make informed decisions about their own health care. They offer a number of clinical practice guidelines on common health problems in consumer versions for the public.

American College of Surgeons (ACoS)
Commission on Cancer
633 North Saint Clair Street
Chicago, IL 60611-3211
Phone: 312-202-5000;
312-202-5085 Cancer Programs
Fax: 312-202-5009 or 5011
Web site: *http://www.facs.org*

The ACoS Commission on Cancer accredits cancer programs of health care organizations in the United States. This voluntary approval program includes a site visit to evaluate the program's compliance with specific standards in ten major areas—from prevention to end-of-life care.

National Cancer Data Base (NCDB)
Web site: *http://www.facs.org/dept/cancer/ncdb*

The NCDB is a nationwide oncology outcomes database for close to 1,500 health care facilities with approved cancer programs in 50 states. It is estimated that close to 80 percent of newly diagnosed cases of cancer are submitted annually to the NCDB, which is jointly supported by the ACS and the ACoS Commission on Cancer.

American Institute for Cancer Research (AICR)
1759 R Street NW
Washington, DC 20009
Toll-Free: 800-843-8114
Phone: 202-328-7744
Fax: 202-328-7226
Web site: *http://www.aicr.org*

The AICR supports research into the role of diet and nutrition in the prevention and treatment of cancer. It also offers a wide range of cancer education programs and publications for health professionals and the public.

Cancer Research Institute (CRI)
681 Fifth Avenue
New York, NY 10022
Toll-Free: 800-99-CANCER (800-992-2623)
Phone: 212-688-7515
Fax: 212-688-7515
Web site: *http://www.cancerresearch.org*

CRI supports research aimed at developing new immunologic methods of diagnosing, treating, and preventing cancer. CRI can answer questions about cancer immunology and provide assistance in locating clinical trials studying immunotherapy.

Centers for Disease Control and Prevention (CDC)

Public Inquiries/MASO
MS F07
1600 Clifton Road NE
Atlanta, GA 30333
Phone: 404-639-3534
Toll-free: 800-311-3435
Web site: *http://www.cdc.gov*

The CDC is an agency of the U.S. Department of Health and Human Services (HHS; see page 244). Their mission is to promote health and quality of life by preventing and controlling disease, injury, and disability. Their Web site contains a searchable map of the 12 centers, offices, and institutes, information about health topics, downloadable publications, and links to related sources.

Federal Trade Commission (FTC)

Consumer Response Center
Federal Trade Commission
CRC-240
Washington, DC 20580
Phone: 877-FTC-HELP (877-382-4357) (toll free); 202-326-2222
Web site: *http://www.ftc.gov*

The Web site includes a Consumer Protection section (available from the home page) where information can be found on topics including health and fitness and consumer fraud.

Food and Agriculture Organization of the United Nations (FAO)

Viale delle Terme di Caracalla, 00100
Rome, Italy
Phone: +39 06 5705 1
Fax: +39 06 5705 3152
Telex: 625852/610181 FAO I /
Web site: *http://www.fao.org*

The FAO of the United Nations was founded in 1945 with a mandate to raise levels of nutrition and standards of living, to improve agricultural productivity, and to better the condition of rural populations. Today, FAO is one of the largest specialized agencies in the United Nations system and the lead agency for agriculture, forestry, fisheries, and rural development. The FAO Web site includes information about nutrition and food safety and quality.

The Mautner Project

1707 L Street NW, Suite 230
Washington, DC 20036
Phone: 202-332-5536
Fax: 202-332-0662
E-mail: mautner@mautnerproject.org
Web site: *http://www.mautnerproject.org*

This organization provides direct services, navigation, and support to lesbians with cancer, their families, and caregivers; education and information to the lesbian community about cancer; education to the health-providing community about the special concerns of lesbians with cancer and their families; and advocacy for lesbian health and cancer issues in national and local arenas. *Some brochures are also available in Spanish. A Spanish Web site is available at http://www.mautnerproject.org/spanish.html.*

National Cancer Institute (NCI)

NCI Public Inquiries Office
Building 31, Room 10A31
31 Center Drive, MSC 2580
Bethesda, MD 20892-2580
Toll-Free: 800-4-CANCER (800-422-6237)
Web site: *http://www.cancer.gov*

This government agency, as part of the National Institutes of Health (NIH; see page 242) provides information on cancer research, diagnosis, and treatment through several services (see the following list). People with cancer, caregivers, and health care professionals may call the NCI's toll-free telephone service for cancer-related information. Includes information about complementary and alternative medicine and nutrition in cancer care. *Spanish-speaking staff and Spanish materials are available.*

CancerFax

Toll-Free Fax: 800-624-2511
Fax: 301-402-5874

CancerFax includes information about cancer treatment, screening, prevention, and supportive care. To obtain a contents list, dial the fax number from a fax machine hand set and follow the recorded instructions.

Cancer Information Service (CIS)

Toll-Free: 800-4-CANCER (800-422-6237)
Toll-Free (TTY): 800-332-8615
Web site: *http://cis.nci.nih.gov*

The CIS provides information to consumers and health care professionals. The Web site contains a wealth of information including pamphlets and brochures on cancer diagnosis, treatment, research, and prevention. *Spanish-speaking staff is available.*

CancerNet

Web site: *http://cancernet.gov*
Web site (Spanish version):
http://cancernet.gov/sp_menu.htm
Web site (on-line ordering):
http://publications.nci.nih.gov

CancerNet is a comprehensive Web site that contains information on diagnosis, treatment, support, resources, literature, clinical trials, prevention and risk factors, and testing. Up to twenty publications can be ordered on-line. The publications list is searchable. *Some publications are available in Spanish.*

Office of Cancer Complementary and Alternative Medicine (OCCAM)

National Cancer Institute, NIH
6116 Executive Plaza North
Suite 600, MSC 8339
Bethesda, MD 20852
Toll-free: 888-NIH-NCAM (888-644-6226) for the National Center for Complementary and Alternative Medicine (NCCAM) Clearinghouse
Web site: *http://www3.cancer.gov/occam*

The OCCAM coordinates and enhances the activities of the NCI in the arena of complementary and alternative medicine. The goal of the OCCAM is to increase the amount of high-quality cancer research and information about the use of complementary and alternative modalities.

National Consumers League

1701 K Street NW, Suite 1201
Washington, DC 20006
Phone: 202-835-3323
Fax: 202-835-0747
Web site: *http://www.nclnet.org*

Experts in law, business, and labor provide consumer protection and advocacy. The National Consumers League publishes educational brochures about general health issues, including cancer-screening tests.

National Council Against Health Fraud

119 Foster Street
Peabody, MA 01960
Phone: 978-532-9383
Web site: *http://www.ncahf.org*

This private, nonprofit voluntary health agency focuses on health misinformation, fraud, and quackery, and provides information on unusual methods of cancer management. It can refer people to lawyers and help those who have had negative experiences to share their story.

National Institutes of Health (NIH)

9000 Rockville Pike
Bethesda, MD 20892
Mailing address:
NIH Building 1
1 Center Drive
Bethesda, Maryland 20892
Toll-free: 800-4-CANCER (800-422-6237);
(TYY) 800-332-8615
Phone: 301-496-4000
Web site: *http://www.nih.gov*

The NIH is one of the world's foremost medical research centers, and the federal focal point for medical research in the United States. The NIH, comprised of 27 separate Institutes and Centers, is one of the eight health agencies of the Public Health Service, which, in turn, is part of the U.S. Department of Health and Human Services (HHS; see page 244). The goal of NIH research is to acquire new knowledge to help prevent, detect, diagnose, and treat disease and disability, from the rarest genetic disorder to the common cold. The NIH mission is to uncover new knowledge that will lead to better health for everyone. (See also the Office of Dietary Supplements, page 245.)

National Center for Complementary and Alternative Medicine (NCCAM)

NCCAM Clearinghouse
P.O. Box 8218
Silver Spring, MD 20907-8218
Toll-free: 888-644-6226; (TYY) 866-464-3615
Phone: 301-231-7537, ext. 5 (from outside the U.S.)
Fax: 301-495-4957
Web site: *http://nccam.nih.gov*

This center provides research-based information on complementary and alternative methods being promoted to treat different diseases, including research and an up-to-date listing of clinical trials on alternative medicine.

The National Institute of Environmental Health Sciences (NIEHS)
P.O. Box 12233
Research Triangle Park, NC 27709
Phone: 919-541-3345; (TTY) 919-541-0731
Web site: *http://www.niehs.nih.gov*

The mission of the NIEHS is to reduce the burden of human illness and dysfunction from environmental causes by understanding environmental factors, individual susceptibility, and age and how they interrelate. The NIEHS achieves its mission through multidisciplinary biomedical research programs, prevention and intervention efforts, and communication strategies that encompass training, education, technology transfer, and community outreach.

National Library of Medicine (NLM)
8600 Rockville Pike
Bethesda, MD 20894
Toll-free: 888-FIND-NLM (888-346-3656)
for the Reference and Customer Service
Telephone Desk
Phone: 301-594-5983
Fax: 301-402-1384
Web site: *http://www.nlm.nih.gov*

The NLM collects, organizes, and makes available biomedical science information to investigators, educators, and practitioners and carries out programs designed to strengthen medical library services in the United States. Its electronic databases are used extensively throughout the world by both health professionals and the public. *Materials are available in languages other than English.*

Internet Grateful Med
Web site: *http://igm.nlm.nih.gov*

This Internet-based service provides access to millions of literature references and abstracts in MEDLINE and other databases, with links to on-line journals. The site is searchable by keywords.

MEDLINEplus
Web site: *http://www.nlm.nih.gov/medlineplus/medlineplus*

MEDLINEplus is a database for consumer health information including dictionaries; articles and journals from other organizations; textbooks, newsletters, and health news for on-line reading; and links to organizations that provide consumer information and clearinghouses that send health literature.

NLM Gateway
Web site: *http://gateway.nlm.nih.gov/gw/Cmd*

The NLM Gateway offers links to searchable databases and allows users to search simultaneously in multiple retrieval systems.

PubMed
Web site: *http://www.ncbi.nlm.nih.gov/PubMed*

This database provides access to millions of literature references and abstracts in MEDLINE and other databases, with links to on-line journals. The site is searchable by keyword.

Women's Health Initiative (WHI)
Women's Health Initiative Program Office
1 Rockledge Centre
Suite 300, MS 7966
6705 Rockledge Drive
Bethesda, MD 20892-7966 (U.S. Postal Service)
Bethesda, MD 20817-7966 (Express Mail Service)
Phone: 301-402-2900
Fax: 301-480-5158
Web site: *http://www.nhlbi.nih.gov/whi/index.html*

The WHI, the largest clinical trial ever undertaken in the United States, addresses the most common causes of death, disability, and impaired quality of life in postmenopausal women. It is expected that the WHI will provide many answers concerning possible benefits and risks associated with use of hormone replacement therapy, dietary supplements, and other interventions in preventing cardiovascular disease, breast and colorectal cancer, and osteoporosis in postmenopausal women.

United States Department of Health and Human Services (HHS)
200 Independence Avenue SW
Washington, DC 20201
Toll Free: 877-696-6775
Phone: 202-619-0257
Web site: *http://www.hhs.gov*

The Department of Health and Human Services (HHS) is the U.S. government's principal agency for protecting the health of all Americans and providing essential human services, especially for those who are least able to help themselves. One of the largest federal agencies, the HHS' responsibilities include public health (CDC, NIH, FDA, and others included), biomedical research, and more. Includes information about the Department of Health and Human Services' Good Manufacturing Processes, or GMPs, being developed by which dietary supplements must be manufactured.

United States Environmental Protection Agency (EPA)
Ariel Rios Building
1200 Pennsylvania Avenue NW
Washington, DC 20460
Phone: 202-260-2090
Web site: *http://www.epa.gov*

The EPA implements the federal laws designed to promote public health by protecting our nation's air, water, and soil from harmful pollution. The Web site offers environmental news, community concerns, information about laws and other regulations, and links to other sources of information.

Office of Pesticide Programs (OPP)
Web site: *http://www.epa.gov/pesticides*

The mission of the OPP is to protect public health and the environment from the risks posed by pesticides and to promote safer means of pest control. The Web site provides consumer alerts, information about pesticides and their use and disposal, a kid's section, industry-related topics, and other information.

Office of Water (OW)
Safe Drinking Water Hotline: 800-426-4791
Web site: *http://www.epa.gov/water*

The OW is responsible for the EPA's water quality activities, including development of national programs, technical policies, and regulations relating to drinking water, water quality, ground water, pollution source standards, and the protection of wetlands, marine, and estuarine areas.

Water Quality Association (WQA)
4151 Naperville Road
Lisle, IL 60532-1088
Phone: 630-505-0160
Fax: 630-505-9637
E-mail: info@wqa.org
Web site: *http://www.wqa.org/*

The WQA is a trade association representing the household, commercial, industrial, and small community water treatment industry. WQA is a resource and information source, a voice for the industry, an educator for professionals, a laboratory for product testing, and a communicator to the public.

World Health Organization (WHO)
WHO Headquarters
Avenue Appia 20
1211 Geneva 27
Switzerland
Telephone: +41 22 791 2111
Facsimile (fax): +41 22 791 3111
United States Headquarters:
Regional Office for the Americas/Pan American Health Organization
525 23rd Street NW
Washington, DC 20037
Phone: 202-974-3000; 202-974-3457 for the Office of Public Information
Fax: 202-974-3663
Web site: *http://www.who.int*

Founded in 1948, the WHO leads the world alliance for Health for All. A specialized agency of the United Nations, WHO promotes technical cooperation for health among nations, carries out programs to control and eradicate disease, and strives to improve the quality of human life.

Organizations Providing Health, Food, Diet, and Supplement Information

American Dietetic Association (ADA)
216 West Jackson Boulevard, Suite 800
Chicago, IL 60606-6995
Phone: 312-899-0040
Web site: *http://www.eatright.org*

The ADA is the world's largest organization of food and nutrition professionals. The ADA serves the public by promoting nutrition, health, and well-being. The Web site contains information on diet and nutrition, publications, and a registered dietitian locator service, including access to dietitians who specialize in oncology nutrition.

International Food Information Council (IFIC) Foundation
1100 Connecticut Avenue NW, Suite 430
Washington, DC 20036
Phone: 202-296-6540
Fax: 202-296-6547
E-mail: foodinfo@ific.org
Web site: *http://ific.org*

As the educational arm of the IFIC, the IFIC Foundation communicates science-based information on food safety and nutrition to health and nutrition professionals, educators, journalists, and others for distribution to consumers. The IFIC has established partnerships with a wide range of professional organizations and academic institutions to develop science-based information for the public.

Meals on Wheels Association of America (MOWAA)
1414 Prince Street, Suite 302
Alexandria, VA 22314
Phone: 703-548-5558
Fax: 703-548-8024
Web site: *http://www.mowaa.org*

Meals on Wheels is a membership association of programs that provide home-delivered and group meals. The goal of the organization is to improve the quality of life of the needy, particularly the elderly, disabled, and homebound. Some programs may provide other health and social services such as transportation, recreation, nutrition, education, information, referrals, and case management.

Memorial Sloan-Kettering Cancer Center (MSKCC)
AboutHerbs
http://www.mskcc.org/mskcc/html/11570.cfm

Memorial Sloan-Kettering Cancer Center's AboutHerbs Web site provides information for consumers about herbs, botanicals, and alternative or unproven cancer therapies, including details about adverse effects, interactions, and potential benefits or problems.

The Office of Dietary Supplements (ODS)
National Institutes of Health
6100 Executive Blvd., Room 3B01, MSC 7517
Bethesda, Maryland 20892-7517
Phone: 301-435-2920
Fax: 301-480-1845
E-mail: ods@nih.gov
Web site: *http://dietary-supplements.info.nih.gov*

The ODS supports research and shares research results about dietary supplements. To explore the role of dietary supplements in the improvement of health care, the ODS plans, organizes, and supports conferences, workshops, and symposia on scientific topics related to dietary supplements.

Quackwatch
Web site: *http://www.quackwatch.com*

Quackwatch is a nonprofit corporation whose purpose is to combat health-related frauds, myths, fads, and fallacies.

United States Department of Agriculture (USDA)
Fourteenth and Independence Avenue SW
Washington, DC 20250-9410
Phone: 202-720-2791
Web site: *http://www.usda.gov*

The USDA strives to enhance the quality of life for the American people by supporting production of agriculture. The USDA is also responsible for the food supply, managing agricultural products, forests, and rangeland, and community development.

The Interactive Healthy Eating Index (IHEI)
Web site: *http://147.208.9.133/Default.asp*

This online dietary assessment tool is based on the Healthy Eating Index developed by the USDA's Center for Nutrition Policy and Promotion. It includes nutrition messages and links to nutrient information.

USDA Food and Nutrition Information Center (FNIC)
National Agricultural Library, Room 304
10301 Baltimore Avenue
Beltsville, MD 20705-2351
Phone: 301-504-5719; 301-504-5414 (for inquiries to dietitians and nutritionists)
Fax: 301-504-6409
E-mail: fnic@nal.usda.gov
Web site: *http://www.nal.usda.gov/fnic*

The USDA's FNIC is an information center for the National Agricultural Library. FNIC materials and services include dietitians and nutritionists available to answer inquiries, publications on food and nutrition, and resource lists and bibliographies. The FNIC Web site includes information on dietary supplements, food safety, dietary guidelines, food composition facts (including fast food), a list of available publications, and information on popular topics.

United States Food and Drug Administration (FDA)
5600 Fishers Lane
Rockville, MD 20857-0001
Phone: 888-INFO-FDA (888-463-6332)
Fax: 301-443-9767
Web site: *http://www.fda.gov*

The FDA is an agency within the U.S. Department of Health and Human Services (HHS; see page 244) and consists of eight centers/offices. The FDA is a public health agency charged with protecting Americans by enforcing the Federal Food, Drug, and Cosmetic Act and other laws, promoting health by helping safe and effective products reach the market in a timely manner, and monitoring products for continued safety after they are in use. The FDA regulates food, cosmetics, medicines, biologics, medical devices, and radiation-emitting consumer products, as well as feed and drugs for pets and farm animals. The Web site has extensive information about all the products the FDA regulates.

Center for Food Safety and Applied Nutrition (CFSAN) Outreach and Information Center
5100 Paint Branch Parkway (HFS-555)
College Park, MD 20740
Toll-free: 888-SAFEFOOD (888-723-3366); TYY: 800-877-8339
Web site: *http://www.cfsan.fda.gov*

The goal of the Outreach and Information Center is to enhance CFSAN's ability to provide and respond to the public's desire and demand for more useful, timely, and accurate information regarding its regulated products. In addition to providing food safety information, the Outreach and Information Center provides assistance with other CFSAN issues, including nutrition, dietary supplements, food labeling, cosmetics, food additives, and food biotechnology.

United States Pharmacopeial Convention (USP)
12601 Twinbrook Parkway
Rockville, MD 20852
Phone: 800-822-8772
Web site: *http://www.usp.org/*

The USP is an organization dedicated to producing quality control standards for the strength, quality, and purity of pharmaceuticals. In 1997, the USP began publishing standards for dietary supplements. These standards focus on the strength, quality, purity, packaging, and labeling of dietary supplements and are updated yearly.

Glossary

Adequate Intake (AI): The AI is established based on observations about the nutrient when taken by a group of healthy people and is established when a *Recommended Daily Allowance (RDA)* cannot be determined.

adjuvant: along with or after another type of therapy.

alkaloids: organic substances in plants.

allium: a compound in foods such as garlic, shallots, and onions that may have a strong protective effect against prostate cancer.

alternative treatments: treatments that are promoted to replace conventional treatment but are unproven because they have not been scientifically tested, or were tested and found to be ineffective.

amino acids: organic compounds found in plants and animals and are the main components of *protein*.

androgens: the male sex *hormones*; treatment to block their production slows the growth and division of prostate cancer cells.

anemia: a lower than normal red blood cell count.

angiogenesis: the formation of new blood vessels.

anorexia: loss of appetite, which can lead to severe weight loss.

anticoagulant: a drug that prevents or treats blood clotting problems. Also called a *blood thinner*.

antiemetics: medications that provide relief from nausea and vomiting.

antiestrogens: substances (for example, the drug tamoxifen) that block the effects of estrogen in tumor cells, used to treat cancers that depend on *estrogen* for growth.

anti-inflammatory: a drug that reduces pain in and swelling of body tissue.

antigen: a substance on a cell that causes the *immune system* to react, producing an immune response.

antioxidants: a compound—such as natural or synthetic vitamins A, C, and E, *carotenoids*, and many other *phytochemicals*—that blocks the action of activated oxygen molecules, known as *free radicals*, which can damage healthy cells. Brightly colored vegetables and fruits are rich food sources of antioxidants.

apoptosis: programmed cell death.

beta-carotene: one of several *carotenoid antioxidants*; found in many foods that are orange in color and in some green leafy vegetables; converted to *vitamin A* by the body.

biologic therapy: see *immunotherapy*.

blood thinner: a drug that prevents or treats blood clotting problems. Also called an *anticoagulant*.

Body Mass Index (BMI): a table of calculated heights and weights used to help determine if a person is at a healthy weight or may weigh too much.

botanical supplements: supplements made from plants. See also *dietary supplements*.

bran: the outer layer of a grain or seed that is an edible source of *fiber*. See also *whole grains*.

caffeine: a mild stimulant found in coffee, some soft drinks, tea, and in some medications.

calcium: a *mineral* vital for biological processes in the body—especially in maintaining bone density—found naturally in milk, other dairy products, and leafy green vegetables; other foods may be fortified with calcium.

calorie: a measurement of the energy your body gets from food to "fuel" all of its functions, such as breathing, circulating the blood, and physical activity.

cancer: a group of many related diseases, all of which involve the out-of-control growth and spread of abnormal cells.

cancer vaccines: a form of *immunotherapy* involving the use of cancer cells, parts of cells, or pure *antigens*. The vaccine increases the body's response against cancer cells in the body in order to bring about resistance to or to prevent the development of *cancer*.

carbohydrates: breads, pasta, grains, beans, fruits, and vegetables are all sources of carbohydrates, which provide the body with a quick source of *calories* that allow it to function and create heat. See also *complex carbohydrates* and *simple carbohydrates*.

carcinogen: a cancer-causing substance.

carotenoids: these *antioxidants* give many fruits and vegetables their color and are promoted as anti-cancer agents.

catechins: *antioxidants* found in green tea; thought to act as anticancer agents when taken in at high levels.

chemopreventive agents: substances that prevent the development of *cancer* by repairing damaged cells.

chemotherapy: drugs designed to kill cancer cells; most are taken by mouth or injected into the bloodstream.

claims of well being: unevaluated claims about a dietary factor such as *dietary supplements*. These claims do not require the approval of the United States Food and Drug Administration. See also *function claims* or *structure claims* and *health claims*.

clinical trials: medical research studies that determine whether a new treatment is effective and safe for humans.

complementary therapies: methods used to complement, or add to, *proven treatments* rather than to cure disease. They may help control symptoms and improve well-being.

complex carbohydrates: also called starches, complex carbohydrates such as vegetables, nuts, seeds, legumes, and whole grains are an important source of food energy, *fiber*, and key *vitamins* and *minerals*. See also *carbohydrates* and *simple carbohydrates*.

copper: a *trace element* found naturally in foods that assists in the regulation of blood pressure and heart rate and the absorption of iron in the body.

corticosteroids: steroid substances related to hormones produced by the adrenal glands; corticosteroid medication is sometimes used as an anticancer treatment or to reduce persistent nausea.

cruciferous vegetable: a plant, such as broccoli or cauliflower, that contains certain chemicals that may reduce the risk of *cancer*.

cytotoxicity: cell-destroying ability.

Daily Values (DV): numbers on current nutrition labels that show the percentage of a nutrient a person gets by eating one serving of the labeled food. DV are based on *U.S. Recommended Daily Allowances* for people eating 2,000 *calories* per day. See also *Recommended Daily Allowances* and *Adequate Intake*.

dehydration: when the body loses too much water to function well. Severe *diarrhea*, vomiting, excess urination, or high fever may cause dehydration.

diarrhea: the passage of loose or watery stools three or more times a day that occurs when water in the intestine is not reabsorbed back into the body.

diet: the foods you eat and drink, both liquids and solids.

Dietary Reference Intakes (DRIs): the current *Recommended Daily Allowances* are being replaced and expanded with DRIs, which will provide recommended *nutrient* intakes for each gender and for people at different life stages. DRIs include *Recommended Daily Allowance, Adequate Intake, Tolerable Upper Intake Level,* and *Estimated Average Requirement.*

Dietary Supplement Health and Safety Act (DSHEA): gives the Federal Drug Administration permission to stop production of a *dietary supplement* when the FDA proves that the product poses a significant risk to the health of Americans.

dietary supplements: products such as concentrated foodstuffs, *vitamins, minerals, herbal supplements,* and *hormones.* Particularly in the case of people undergoing treatment for cancer, self-medication with dietary supplements may pose health risks.

dietitian: see *registered dietitian.*

digestive tract: the parts of the body involved with eating, digesting, and excreting food, including the mouth, esophagus, stomach, intestines, rectum, and anus.

distillation: a water treatment process that turns water into a vapor. Since *minerals* are too heavy to vaporize, they are left behind.

diuretic: a medication or food that increases urination.

electrolyte: salt and *minerals* in the body important in metabolic activities and in the normal functioning of cells.

endosperm: a seed's source of energy; the nutritional tissues in the seeds of flowering plants. See also *whole grains.*

enteral feeding: see *tube feeding.*

epidemiological study: a type of human study that examines the frequency, distribution, and causes of diseases in large groups of people. The two general categories of epidemiological studies are *observational studies* and *interventional studies.*

essential nutrient: a substance that must be obtained from the diet because the body cannot make enough of it to meet its needs.

Estimated Average Requirement (EAR): the amount of a *nutrient* that is estimated to meet the *nutrition* requirements of half of all healthy individuals in the population.

estrogen: a female sex *hormone* produced primarily by the ovaries that may contribute to the development of some *cancers,* such as breast cancer.

estrogen receptors: molecules on cells that attract *estrogen* circulating in the blood, allowing estrogen to affect the functioning of those cells. Estrogen receptor positive cancers are more likely to respond to *hormonal therapy* than breast cancer cells without these receptors, called estrogen receptor negative cancers.

fat soluble: nutrients such as vitamins A, D, E, and K that are stored by the body in its fat stores. See also *water soluble.*

fats: soft-solid or liquid material found in animal tissues and many plants, made up of *fatty acids* and *calories;* called *saturated, monounsaturated,* or *polyunsaturated,* depending on the type of fatty acids it contains. Fats provide energy for physical activity, produce *hormones,* transport some *vitamins,* and build new cells. The role of fat in cancer risk is controversial and continues to be studied.

fatty acids: derived from *fats,* these are the most concentrated form of calories (energy); they help the body grow, produce *hormones,* transport some *vitamins,* and build new cells. There are three main types of fatty acids: *saturated fatty acids, monounsaturated fatty acids,* and *polyunsaturated fatty acids.* See also *trans fatty acids.*

fiber: the part of plant foods the body cannot digest, which helps to move food waste out of the body quickly. Fiber is found in fruits, vegetables, dry beans and peas, nuts and seeds, and breads and cereals. See also *soluble fiber* and *insoluble fiber.*

flavonoids: *phytochemicals* called *polyphenols,* flavonoids are found in a broad range of grains, vegetables, and fruits, some of which may mimic the actions of *estrogen.*

flaxseed and flaxseed oil: seeds and oil from the flax plant promoted as a dietary *nutrient* with potential *antiestrogen* activity.

folate: see *folic acid.*

folic acid: a *vitamin* (also called vitamin B9) that influences growth, reproduction, blood-cell production, and the nervous system; contained in green leafy vegetables, liver, citrus fruits, mushrooms, nuts, peas, dried beans, and fortified wheat bread.

food additive: any substance used in the production, processing, treatment, packaging, transportation, or storage of food. See also *indirect food additive.*

free radicals: unstable oxygen-free compounds created during normal cell *metabolism* that can damage important cell proteins and enzymes and can cause DNA changes that can contribute to the development of cancer. See also *antioxidants.*

function claims: also called *structure claims*, these are implied benefits of a dietary factor such as *dietary supplements* on body processes; they may appear on food and supplement labels. See also *health claims* and *claims of well-being.*

functional foods: foods modified, bred, fortified, or bioengineered to offer health benefits; also called *nutraceuticals.*

gastrostomy: surgical placement of a tube through the skin into the stomach for the administration of liquid feedings.

genetically modified food: food changed in the laboratory to make it resistant to pests and disease, to increase its concentration of *nutrients*, or to increase quality or shelf life.

germ: the seed, bud, or spore of a new plant. See also *whole grains.*

glucosinolate: a type of *phytochemical* found in many *cruciferous vegetables.*

glycemic index: a way of classifying foods that measures how quickly and how highly a person's blood sugar level rises after eating a food; *carbohydrates* are the highest foods on the glycemic index. See also *high-glycemic foods, insulin,* and *low-glycemic foods.*

Good Manufacturing Processes (GMPs): the set of standards being developed by the Department of Health and Human Services to be used in the manufacturing of *dietary supplements* to prevent their contamination and ensure high quality.

green tea: a drink made from the steamed and dried leaves of the *Camellia sinesis* plant, a shrub native to Asia. Green tea is thought to contain chemicals known as *polyphenols*, which have *antioxidant* and other disease-preventative properties.

health claims: specific claims about the direct effects of a dietary factor, for example, dietary supplements, on the body. See also *structure claims* or *function claims* and *claims of well-being.*

herbal supplements: an entire plant or combination of plants or leaves, roots, or other parts that are sold dried, finely chopped, powdered, in capsule or liquid form. Herbal supplements contain many chemical ingredients, some helpful and others potentially dangerous.

herbal tea: made from different plants than green or black tea and often contain fruit and spices instead of tea leaves; herbal teas do not usually contain the *antioxidants* found in green tea.

herbicide: a chemical that kills weeds.

herbs: taken from plants, the two general groups of herbs are culinary herbs used in cooking to season food and medicinal herbs used as remedies to treat illness, as in *herbal supplements.*

high-glycemic foods: foods (such as highly processed *carbohydrates*, in which the *bran* and *germ* layers are removed) that break down and cause fast, significant increases in a person's blood sugar levels. See also *glycemic index* and *low-glycemic foods.*

hormonal therapy: drug treatment that interferes with *hormone* production or action, or the surgical removal of hormone-producing glands. Hormonal therapy may kill *cancer* cells or slow their growth.

hormone: a chemical substance released by the endocrine glands that travels through the bloodstream to set in motion various body functions.

human study: see *epidemiological study, observational study, interventional study,* and *clinical trial.*

immune system: the complex system by which the body resists infection by microbes (such as bacteria or viruses) and rejects transplanted tissues or organs. The immune system may also help the body fight some cancers.

immunosuppression: weakening of the *immune system*.

immunotherapy: a treatment that stimulates a person's *immune system*. Also called *biologic therapy* or biologic response modifiers.

indirect food additive: a substance that becomes part of food in trace amounts due to its packaging, storage, or other handling. See also *food additive*.

insoluble fiber: dietary fiber not dissolvable in water; examples include wheat bran and cellulose. See also *fiber* and *soluble fiber*.

insulin: a *hormone* naturally produced by the pancreas that allows the body to use glucose (sugar) from food as an energy source.

insulin-like growth factor (IGF): a *hormone* involved in hormone-dependent *cancers* such as breast and prostate cancer. IGF levels are high in people with these cancers.

interventional study: a human study in which researchers intentionally change at least one factor they believe is related to the risk of a disease and then monitor any changes in the disease over time. See also *randomized controlled clinical trial* and *observational study*.

investigational treatments: therapies being studied in a *clinical trial*; not proven.

iron: an essential mineral involved in oxygen transport; found in red meat and in plants such as lentils, beans, as well as in products enriched or fortified with iron, such as cereal. A lack of iron may cause *anemia*.

irradiated food: food which has had harmful organisms killed by radiation in order to extend its shelf life.

isoflavones: found mainly in soybeans; sometimes called *phytoestrogens*, or plant estrogens. These compounds act like weak forms of *estrogens* but are not produced by the body. Genistein and daidzein are two soy isoflavones.

laboratory study: in this type of early stage study, researchers test substances on bacteria, animal, or human cells grown in laboratory dishes or test tubes.

lactase: an enzyme that breaks down the milk sugar *lactose*. See also *lactose intolerance*.

lactose: milk sugar. See also *lactose intolerance*.

lactose intolerance: a state in which the body does not produce enough *lactase* to break down *lactose*, which remains in the intestine. The fermentation of lactose in the bowel causes the formation of gases and can cause *diarrhea* and cramping.

leukocytes: the medical term for white blood cells.

leukopenia: a decreased number of white blood cells; may result from *cancer* treatment.

lignans: compounds that can act as *antiestrogens* or as weak *estrogens*, which may play a role in preventing estrogen-dependent cancers such as breast *cancer* and other cancers.

liquid diet: a clear liquid diet is a short-term dietary plan that includes only about 500 *calories* a day from clear, drinkable liquid (such as apple or cranberry juice, clear broth, and Popsicles) and does not supply adequate *nutrients* for long-term health.

liquid nutrition supplements: drinks used to augment the diet if inadequate *nutrition* is an issue by providing *calories*, *protein*, *vitamins*, and *minerals*. See also *meal replacements*.

low-glycemic foods: foods such as *whole grains*, high-protein, or fat-containing foods that contain unrefined or *complex carbohydrates*, take longer to digest, and raise blood levels more slowly and less than processed foods. See also *glycemic index* and *high-glycemic foods*.

lutein: this *antioxidant* associated with improved eye health is abundant in green, leafy vegetables such as collard greens, spinach, and kale.

lycopene: the compound that gives tomatoes their color and may also have anticancer effects.

lymph nodes: bean-sized collections of *immune system* cells that are scattered throughout the body; they work to remove cell waste and fluids, help fight infection, and play a role in fighting *cancer*.

macrobiotic diet: a dietary regimen that involves eating *whole grains*, vegetables and fruits, soups, occasional fish, and tea; may lack essential *nutrients*.

magnesium: a mineral found in fish, *whole grains*, nuts, and leafy green vegetables that helps bones form and reduces the risk of osteoporosis, builds *protein*, and converts food to energy.

meal replacements: substances that boost or support nutrition when you can't eat enough *calories* or *nutrients* through regular meals or food intake, but should not be a permanent substitute for whole foods.

megadosing: the practice of using large doses of *vitamins*, *minerals*, or other *supplements* to attack disease; this practice can be dangerous.

metabolic therapy: involves using a combination of special diets and other nutritional *supplements* in an attempt to remove "toxins" from the body and strengthen the body's defenses against disease. It is based on the theory that disease is caused by toxic substances that have accumulated in the body.

metabolism: the complex physical and chemical processes occurring within a cell that maintain life; the process of breaking down and building up of molecules to make energy for the body.

micronutrient: a dietary element, such as a *vitamin* or *mineral*, essential in small quantities for growth and health.

minerals: inorganic (neither animal nor vegetable) substances or *nutrients* needed in small amounts by the body to help it function properly and stay strong, such as *iron*, *calcium*, *potassium*, and *sodium*.

molybdenum: a *mineral* involved in many important biological processes. Common sources include legumes, cereals, leafy vegetables, liver, and milk.

monoclonal antibodies: *proteins* produced in the laboratory rather than by the *immune system*; used to deliver treatment directly to *cancer* cells or to help detect and classify cancer cells.

monounsaturated fatty acids: mostly found in plant foods like nuts and olives, monounsaturated fatty acids are believed to lower blood cholesterol. Monounsaturated oils are liquid at room temperature but begin to solidify when refrigerated. See also *fatty acids*.

mucositis: inflammation or ulcerations of a mucous membrane such as the lining of the mouth.

multivitamin/mineral supplement: a pill containing a variety of the *Recommended Daily Allowances* or *Daily Requirements* of *vitamins* and *minerals*.

myelosuppression: insufficient production of blood cells due to suppression of bone marrow activity; may result from *cancer* or cancer treatment.

neutropenia: a shortage of *neutrophils*, a type of white blood cell.

neutrophils: a type of white blood cell that reacts quickly against infection.

nitrites: sodium nitrites are salts added to many meats to maintain color and to prevent contamination with bacteria. Nitrites may be converted in the stomach to carcinogenic nitrosamines, which may increase the risk of stomach *cancer*.

nonspecific immunotherapies: an overall boost to the *immune system* that may result in more activity against any *cancer* cells present.

nutraceutical: any food or food ingredient thought to provide medical or health benefits; a combination of a pharmaceutical nutrient and a nutrition agent; see also *functional food*.

nutrient: chemical compounds, such as *water*, *protein*, *fat*, *carbohydrate*, *vitamins*, and *minerals*, that make up foods and are necessary for human growth and life.

nutrition: a three-part process that gives the body the *nutrients* it needs: eating or drinking food, breaking down the food into nutrients, and the travel of the nutrients through the bloodstream to different parts of the body where they are used for body processes.

Nutrition Facts panel: a label on the side or back of labels of frozen and canned items specifying nutrient content. See also *Percent Daily Value*.

nutritionist: someone who counsels others about food and nutrition. There are no educational requirements associated with the title. See also *registered dietitian*.

observational study: a human study that follows people going about their lives, without any intervention from researchers; used to assess any relationship between lifestyle and demographic factors and disease risk. See also *interventional study*.

omega-3 fatty acids: *polyunsaturated fatty acids* involved in many human biological processes that must be obtained from dietary sources like coldwater fatty fish, flaxseed, or from *supplements*. See also *omega-6 fatty acids*.

omega-6 fatty acids: these fats are found in many vegetable oils (corn, safflower, and sunflower), cereals, snack foods, and baked goods. Omega-6 fats potentially decrease the risk of heart disease but may increase the risk of developing *cancer*. See also *omega-3 fatty acids*.

organic food: often refers to plant foods grown without *pesticides* and *genetic modifications* and is also used to refer to meat, poultry, eggs, and dairy raised without antibiotics or growth *hormones*.

Percent Daily Value: part of the *Nutrition Facts panel* that shows how much a canned or packaged food's level of *nutrients* contribute to the daily *diet*.

pesticides: substances applied to many commercially grown fruit and vegetable crops to help protect them from insects, diseases, weeds, and mold.

phytochemicals: non-nutrient compounds found in fruits, vegetables, beans, grains, and other plants that seem to benefit the body and may even fight *cancer*. Thousands of phytochemicals have been identified; *polyphenols* and *flavonoids* are examples of groups of phytochemicals. Some phytochemicals have either *antioxidant* or *estrogen*-like actions.

phytoestrogens: *estrogen*-like *phytochemicals* found in some plant sources such as soy.

polyphenols: chemicals including *flavonoids* that have *antioxidant* properties.

polyunsaturated fatty acids: mostly found in plant foods like vegetables and grains as well as in some seafood and flaxseed; associated with low blood cholesterol. *Fatty acids* help the body grow, produce *hormones*, transport some *vitamins*, and build new cells. See also *monounsaturated fatty acids* and *saturated fatty acids*.

potassium: a *mineral* that helps regulate major body functions. The body cannot manufacture potassium and must obtain it from foods including apricots, potatoes, bananas, molasses, and orange juice.

progesterone: a female sex *hormone* released by the ovaries during every menstrual cycle. See also *estrogen*.

protein: a *nutrient* that provides the body with *amino acids*, which ensure growth, repair body tissue, maintain a healthy *immune system*, and aid in other body functions. Without enough protein, the body takes longer to recover from illness and lowers its resistance to infection.

proven treatment: evidence-based, or mainstream medical treatments that have been tested following a strict set of guidelines and found to be safe and effective.

radiation therapy: therapy in which radiation—high energy beams—are directed at parts of the body with *cancer* to destroy cancer cells.

randomized controlled clinical trial: an *intervention trial* in which people are randomly assigned to a group that receives an intervention or a control group, which receives no intervention or a different intervention. The goal is to determine if there is a difference in the two groups' outcomes. Randomized controlled clinical trials are the gold standard for study proof.

Recommended Dietary Allowances (RDAs): established by the Food and Nutrition Board; the average daily dietary intake of a *nutrient* that is sufficient to meet the requirement of nearly all (97 to 98 percent of) healthy persons.

recurrence: *cancer* that comes back after treatment, whether in the same place as the original cancer, in the lymph nodes, or after spreading to another area of the body.

refined grains: grains stripped of the *bran* and *germ* during processing that are therefore low in *fiber*, in nutritional value, and in the protective substances that accompany fiber. See also *whole grains*.

registered dietitian (RD): an expert in food and diet who is required to have at least a bachelor's degree, have passed a national competency exam, and continue education throughout his or her career. RDs can help people with *cancer* through dietary counseling and education.

research treatments: therapies being studied in a *clinical trial*.

saturated fatty acids: derived from *fats*, saturated fatty acids raise blood cholesterol. Generally solid at room temperature, they are mostly found in meats and whole-milk products. See also *trans fatty acids*.

secondary cancer: a tumor that forms as a result of *cancer's* spread from its original site or as a result of cancer treatment.

selenium: researchers think this *mineral nutrient* is an *antioxidant*. Selenium may also play a role in normal growth, development, and fertility. The best nutritional sources of selenium are seafood, liver, whole grains, and Brazil nuts.

simple carbohydrates: sugar and honey, which lack the *vitamins*, *minerals*, *proteins*, and *fiber* that are generally found in *complex carbohydrates* but do contribute *calories* (energy) to the diet.

sitz baths: bathing of the hips and buttocks in a warm bath to reduce pain or discomfort in the anal area.

slurry: a mixture of water and a substance; for example, a thin paste of water and flour stirred into a hot dish as a thickener to make the food moist and easier to swallow.

sodium: a *mineral* required to keep body fluids in balance. Sodium is found in table salt. Too much sodium can cause you to retain water and may raise your blood pressure.

soluble fiber: dietary fiber like oat bran that is dissolvable in water and when eaten, helps to reduce blood cholesterol, lowering the risk of coronary heart disease. See also *fiber* and *insoluble fiber*.

soy: tofu, soybeans (edamame), soy milk, and soy powder are all forms of the soybean plant. The *isoflavones* in soy and miso (such as genistein and daidzein) have estrogen-like properties and may possibly play a role in *cancer* risk.

structure claims: also called *function claims*; implied benefits of a dietary factor such as *dietary supplements* on body processes; they may appear on food and supplement labels. See also *health claims* and *claims of well-being*.

sulfides: a group of *phytochemicals* found in garlic and onions being studied for possible preventative or disease-reversing properties.

supplements: see *dietary supplements* and *multivitamin/mineral supplements*.

surgery: *cancer* surgery is a treatment that removes cancer cells and surrounding tissue from the body and is often combined with *radiation therapy* and *chemotherapy* to treat cancer. It also plays an important role in cancer diagnosis and staging (finding out whether cancer has spread and if so, how far).

Tolerable Upper Intake Level (UL): the highest daily intake of a *nutrient* that is likely to be safe for almost all individuals—that is, likely not to pose any risks of toxicity. The risk of side effects increases as the intake above the UL increases.

total parenteral nutrition (TPN): delivery of *nutrients* directly into the bloodstream through a needle inserted into a vein; used when eating is extremely limited or not possible.

trace element: a chemical element, such as *copper* or *zinc*, found in small amounts in the human body that is necessary for body processes.

trans fatty acids: also called trans-saturated fats and trans fats, these fats are not found in nature but are formed by adding hydrogen to polyunsaturated fats to give them longer shelf lives; found in most margarines, vegetable shortenings, and packaged breads, cakes, cookies, and crackers. They are similar to *saturated fat* in that raise blood cholesterol. See also *fatty acids*.

tube feeding: also called *enteral nutrition*; a small, thin, flexible tube placed into the nose or directly into the gastrointestinal tract to provide liquid *nutrients* when a person cannot eat enough.

UL: see *Tolerable Upper Intake Level*.

unproven or untested treatment: sometimes refers to treatments with little basis in scientific fact, but may also refer to treatments or tests that are under scientific investigation.

U.S. Recommended Daily Allowances (U.S. RDAs): based on but not exactly the same as the Food and Nutrition Board's *Recommended Daily Allowances*. The Food and Drug Administration developed the U.S. RDA system in the 1970s. See also *Daily Value*.

vegetarianism: a dietary regimen that involves eating food from plant sources such as vegetables and fruits, grains, legumes, seeds, and nuts. Some vegetarian *diets* include no animal products (vegan), while others include dairy products (lactovegetarian) or dairy and eggs (lacto-ovo-vegetarian).

vitamin A: a vitamin essential for normal growth, bone development, reproduction, healing, and vision; taken in directly as vitamin A from animal sources and taken in indirectly from many fruits and vegetables as beta-carotene, which the body converts to vitamin A.

vitamin B1: a vitamin (also called thiamine) that regulates enzymes that influence the functions of the muscles, nerves, and heart; found in cereals and *whole grains* as well as potatoes, pork, seafood, liver, and kidney beans.

vitamin B2: a vitamin (also called riboflavin) that influences the production of energy in cells and health of the skin and mucous membranes of the digestive and respiratory systems; found in enriched bread, dairy products, liver, and green leafy vegetables.

vitamin B3: a vitamin (also called niacin) that has a role in production of energy in cells and in maintaining health of the skin, nervous system, and digestive system; found in liver, fish, chicken, lean red meat, nuts, *whole grains*, and dried beans.

vitamin B5: a vitamin (also called pantothenic acid) that influences normal growth and development and is found in almost all foods.

vitamin B6: a vitamin (also called pyridoxine) with an effect on *protein*, *carbohydrate*, and *fat* metabolism, and on maintaining health of red blood cells, skin, the nervous system, and the digestive system. Fish, liver, pork, chicken, potatoes, wheat germ, bananas, and dried beans are good sources of vitamin B6.

vitamin B12: a vitamin (also called cobalamin) that plays a role in growth, development, the production of blood cells, the functions of the nervous system, and how the body uses *folic acid* and *carbohydrates*. It is found in meats, fish, eggs, and dairy products.

vitamin C: an essential vitamin that must be obtained from the *diet*, in citrus fruits like oranges, grapefruit, and lemons, and in green leafy vegetables, potatoes, strawberries, bell peppers, and cantaloupe. Vitamin C helps bones and teeth form, helps resist infection, helps wounds heal, and is needed for blood clotting. It is also an *antioxidant*.

vitamin D: a vitamin that maintains normal blood levels of *calcium* and phosphorus. It aids in the absorption of calcium, helping to form and maintain strong bones. Only a few foods naturally contain significant amounts of vitamin D, including fatty fish and fish oils. In the United States, milk is fortified with vitamin D.

vitamin E: an essential *nutrient* that helps build normal cells and form red blood cells. The main sources of vitamin E in the diet are vegetable oils (especially safflower oil, sunflower oil, and cottonseed oil), green leafy vegetables, nuts, cereals, meats, egg yolks, wheat germ, and whole wheat products.

vitamin K: an essential *nutrient* the liver needs to form substances that promote blood clotting and prevent abnormal bleeding. The human body obtains vitamin K from certain foods and bacteria that normally live in the intestines. Dietary sources of vitamin K include leafy greens, as well as cereals, dairy products, some fruits, liver, and pork.

vitamins: key *nutrients*, such as vitamins A, C, and E, that the body needs in small amounts to grow and stay strong and active.

water: water and fluids make up from one half to two thirds of your total body weight. Water regulates the body's temperature, transports *nutrients* where they are needed, and removes waste.

water soluble: *nutrients* that can dissolve in water and that the body cannot store in fat tissues; excess amounts are excreted in the urine. Humans need to take in water soluble nutrients such as vitamins B and C every day. See also *fat soluble*.

whole grains: grains such as barley, brown rice, whole wheat, or bulgur that contain the *germ*, *endosperm*, and *bran* of a grain or seed. Different whole-grain foods differ in *nutrient* content, but they provide more *vitamins*, *minerals*, *fiber*, and other protective substances than *refined grains*.

zinc: zinc (as well as zinc gluconate or zinc sulfate) is a *trace element* that plays a key role in many body processes, including the building of DNA, energy production, cell metabolism, and regulation of the *immune system*. Zinc is found in lean meat, seafood, soybeans, nuts, pumpkin and sunflower seeds, eggs, cheese, and wheat bran.

References

Introduction

Brown, Jean et al. 2001. "Nutrition During and After Cancer Treatment: A Guide for Informed Choices by Cancer Survivors." *CA: A Cancer Journal for Clinicians* 51:153–181 (May/June).

University of Michigan Comprehensive Cancer Center. 2003. "Why It Is Important to Eat Well." Managing Eating Problems. Available at: *http://www.cancer.med. umich.edu/learn/nutreatwell.htm.*

Chapter 1

American Cancer Society. 1998. "The American Cancer Society's Skinny on Trimming the Fat." ACS News Today (24 February). Available at: *http://www.cancer.org/docroot/ MED/content/MED_2_1X_The_American_Cancer_Society_ s_Skinny_on_Trimming_the_Fat.asp.*

American Cancer Society. 2000. *American Cancer Society's Guide to Complementary and Alternative Cancer Methods.* Atlanta, Georgia: American Cancer Society.

American Cancer Society. 2001. "Cancer Patients Want—and Need—Better Nutrition Information." ACS News Today (21 November). Available at: *http://www. cancer.org/ docroot/nws/content/nws_1_1x_cancer_patients_want__and _need__better_nutrition_information.asp.*

American Cancer Society. 2002. *Good for You! Reducing Your Risk of Developing Cancer.* Atlanta, Georgia: American Cancer Society.

American Cancer Society. 2003. "Benefits of Good Nutrition." Available at: *http://www.cancer.org/docroot/ MBC/content/MBC_6_2X_Benefits_of_nutrition_during_ treatment.asp?sitearea=MBC.*

American Institute of Cancer Research. 2002. "Survivors Guide: Understanding the Diet-Cancer Connection." Available at: *http://www.aicr.org/survivor.*

Brown, Jean et al. 2001. "Nutrition During and After Cancer Treatment: A Guide for Informed Choices by Cancer Survivors." *CA: A Cancer Journal for Clinicians* 51:153–181 (May/June).

Brown, Jean et al. 2003. "Nutrition and Physical Activity During and After Cancer Treatment: An American Cancer Society Guide for Informed Choices." *CA: A Cancer Journal for Clinicians* 53:268–291 (September/October).

Frazier, A. Lindsay et al. 2003. "Adolescent Diet and Risk of Breast Cancer." *Breast Cancer Research* 5 (2):R59–64 (21 February).

Ghosh, Kris, Linda Carson, and Elyse Cohen. 2002. *Betty Crocker's Living with Cancer Cookbook.* New York: Hungry Minds.

Kantor, Linda S. et al. 2001. "Choose a Variety of Grains Daily, Especially Whole Grains: A Challenge for Consumers." *The Journal of Nutrition* 131 (2S-1):473S–86S (February).

Kurtzweil, Paula. 2003. "Fruits and Vegetables: Eating Your Way to 5 a Day." *FDA Consumer Magazine.* United States Food and Drug Administration (January). Available at: *http://www.cfsan.fda.gov/~dms/fda5aday.html.*

Margie, Joyce Daly, and Abby S. Bloch. 1984. *Nutrition and the Cancer Patient.* Radnor, Pennsylvania: Chilton Publishing.

Mayfield, Eleanor. 1999. *FDA Consumer Magazine,* "A Consumer's Guide to Fats." United States Food and Drug Administration (January). Available at: *http://vm.cfsan.fda.gov/~dms/fdfats.html.*

McCullough, Marjorie L. et al. 2000. "Adherence to US Dietary Guidelines and Risk of Major Chronic Disease in Women." *American Journal of Clinical Nutrition* 72:1214–22 (November).

National Cancer Institute. 1997. "Eating Hints for Cancer Patients: Before, During, and After Treatment." Available at: *http://www.cancer.gov/cancerinfo/eatinghints*.

Office of the Surgeon General. 2001. "Overweight and Obesity: At a Glance." *The Surgeon General's Call To Action To Prevent and Decrease Overweight and Obesity*. Available at: *http://www.surgeongeneral.gov/topics/obesity/calltoaction/fact_glance.htm*.

Penland, James G. 2002. "Dietary Reference Intakes (DRIs): New Dietary Guidelines Really Are New!" Grand Forks Human Nutrition Research Center. United States Food and Drug Administration. Available at: *http://www.gfhnrc.ars.usda.gov/News/nws9912a.htm*.

United States Food and Drug Administration. 2003. "Answers to Frequently Asked Questions." Food Nutrition and Information Center. Available at: *http://www.nal.usda.gov/fnic/foodcomp/Bulletins/faq.html*.

Chapter 2

American Cancer Society. 2000. *American Cancer Society's Guide to Complementary and Alternative Cancer Methods*. Atlanta, Georgia: American Cancer Society.

Anderson, Jean, and Barbara Deskins. 1995. *The Nutrition Bible: A Comprehensive, No-Nonsense Guide to Foods, Nutrients, Additives, Preservatives, Pollutants and Everything Else We Eat and Drink*. New York: William Morrow and Company, Inc.

Brody, Jane E. 2003. "For Unrefined Healthfulness: Refined Grains." *The New York Times*, Personal Health (4 March).

Brown, Jean et al. 2003. "Nutrition and Physical Activity During and After Cancer Treatment: An American Cancer Society Guide for Informed Choices." *CA: A Cancer Journal for Clinicians* 53:268–291 (September/October).

Erlund, Iris et al. 2003. "Consumption of Black Currants, Lingonberries and Bilberries Increases Serum Quercetin Concentrations." *European Journal of Clinical Nutrition* 57 (1):37–42 (January).

Harvard School of Public Health. 2003. "Carbohydrates." Nutrition Source. Available at: *http://www.hsph.harvard.edu/nutritionsource/carbohydrates.html*.

International Food Information Council Foundation. 2002. "Functional Foods Fact Sheet: Antioxidants." Food Safety and Nutrition Information (June). Available at: *http://ific.org/proactive/newsroom/release.vtml?id=20921*.

Karas, Michael et al. 2000. "Lycopene Interferes with Cell Cycle Progression and Insulin-like Growth Factor I Signaling in Mammary Cancer Cells." *Nutrition and Cancer* 36 (1):101–11 (January).

Kurtzweil, Paula. 1998. *FDA Consumer Magazine*. "Better Information for Special Diets." United States Food and Drug Administration (January). Available at: *http://www.cfsan.fda.gov/~dms/fdspdiet.html*.

Kurtzweil, Paula. 2003. *FDA Consumer Magazine*. "Fruits and Vegetables: Eating Your Way to 5 a Day." United States Food and Drug Administration (January). Available at: *http://www.cfsan.fda.gov/~dms/fda5aday.html*.

Memorial Sloan-Kettering Cancer Center. 2003. AboutHerbs. Information Resource: AboutHerbs, Botanicals & Other Products. Available at: *http://www.mskcc.org/aboutherbs*.

United States Department of Agriculture. 2002. "Dietary Guidelines for Americans: Putting the Guidelines into Practice." *Home and Garden Bulletin No. 267-2*. Center for Nutrition Policy and Promotion (May).

United States Department of Health and Human Services, United States Department of Agriculture. 2000. "Nutrition and Your Health: Dietary Guidelines for Americans." Available at: *http://www.health.gov/dietaryguidelines/dga2000/document/build.htm*.

Chapter 3

Allred, Clinton D. et al. 2001. "Soy Diets Containing Varying Amounts of Genistein Stimulate Growth of Estrogen-Dependent (MCF-7) Tumors in a Dose-Dependent Manner." *Cancer Research* 61: 5045–50 (1 July).

American Cancer Society. 2000. *American Cancer Society's Guide to Complementary and Alternative Cancer Methods*. Atlanta, Georgia: American Cancer Society.

Brown, Jean et al. 2003. "Nutrition and Physical Activity During and After Cancer Treatment: An American Cancer Society Guide for Informed Choices." *CA: A Cancer Journal for Clinicians* 53:268–291 (September/October).

National Cancer Institute. 2002. "Fact Sheet: Red Wine and Cancer Prevention." NCI News Center (27 November). Available at: *http://www.cancer.gov/newscenter/pressreleases/redwine*.

National Cancer Institute. 2002. "Fact Sheet: Tea and Cancer Prevention." NCI News Center (6 December). Available at: *http://www.cancer.gov/newscenter/content_nav.aspx?viewid=afc8f2c0-f3df-4f6c-9c30-28fc15c0054e*.

Tavani, A., and C. La Vecchia. 2000. "Coffee and Cancer: A Review of Epidemiological Studies, 1990–1999." *European Journal of Cancer Prevention* 9 (4):241–256 (August).

University of California at Davis Health System. 2000. "Breast Cancer." *The Well-Connected Report* (March). Available at: *http://wellness.ucdavis.edu/medical_conditions_az/breastcancer06.html*.

World Health Organization. 2003. "Micronutrient Deficiencies: Combating Vitamin A Deficiency" (9 April). Available at: *http://www.who.int/nut/vad.htm*.

Chapter 4
American Cancer Society. 1998. "Souping Up Your Immune System." ACS News Today (24 November). Available at: *http://www.cancer.org/docroot/NWS/content/NWS_1_1x_Souping_Up_Your_Immune_System.asp*.

American Cancer Society. 2002. *Good for You! Reducing Your Risk of Developing Cancer*. Atlanta, Georgia: American Cancer Society.

Anderson, Jean, and Barbara Deskins. 1995. *The Nutrition Bible: A Comprehensive, No-Nonsense Guide to Foods, Nutrients, Additives, Preservatives, Pollutants, and Everything Else We Eat and Drink*. New York: William Morrow and Company.

Brody, Jane E. 2003. "For Unrefined Healthfulness: Refined Grains." *The New York Times* Personal Health (4 March).

Kurtzweil, Paula. 2003. *FDA Consumer Magazine*. "Fruits and Vegetables: Eating Your Way to 5 a Day." United States Food and Drug Administration (January). Available at: *http://www.cfsan.fda.gov/~dms/fda5aday.html*.

New York Times. 2001. "Genetically Modified Organisms." Health: Genetics, Recent Coverage. Available at: *http://www.nytimes.com/library/national/science/health/gm-index.html*.

Nutrition News Focus. 1998. "Pesticides on Fruits and Vegetables" (November).

United States Environmental Protection Agency, Office of Pesticide Programs. 1998. "Pesticides on Food: Consumer Information" (January). Available at: *http://www.epa.gov/fedrgstr/EPA-PEST/1998/January/Day-14/6020.pdf*.

United States General Accounting Office. 2002. "Genetically Modified Foods: Experts View Regimen of Safety Tests as Adequate, but FDA's Evaluation Process Could Be Enhanced" (May). Available at: *http://www.gao.gov/docdblite/summary.php?recflag=&accno=A03410&rptno=GAO-02-566*.

United States Food and Drug Administration. 2001. "Food Additives." Food and Drug Administration/International Food Information Council Brochure (August). Available at: *http://www.cfsan.fda.gov/~lrd/foodaddi.html*.

United States Food and Drug Administration. 2000. "Food Irradiation: A Safe Measure." Publication No. (FDA) 00-2329 (January). Available at: *http://www.fda.gov/opacom/catalog/irradbro.html*.

United States Food and Drug Administration. 2002. "Labeling and Marketing Information." The National Organic Program (October). Available at: *http://www.ams.usda.gov/nop/FactSheets/LabelingE.html*.

United States Food and Drug Administration. 2002. "Organic Food Standards and Labels: The Facts." The National Organic Program (April). Available at: *http://www.ams.usda.gov/nop/Consumers/brochure.html*.

World Health Organization. 2003. "Micronutrient Deficiencies: Combating Vitamin A Deficiency" (9 April). Available at: *http://www.who.int/nut/vad.htm*.

Chapter 5
Agus, David B. et al. 1999. "Stromal Cell Oxidation: A Mechanism by which Tumors Obtain Vitamin C." *Cancer Research* 59 (18): 4555–8 (19 September).

American Cancer Society. 2000. *American Cancer Society's Guide to Complementary and Alternative Cancer Methods*. Atlanta, Georgia: American Cancer Society.

Cyberbotanica. 1997. "Plants and Cancer Treatments." BioTech Resources, Indiana University. Available at: *http://life.nthu.edu.tw/~g864204/botany.html*.

Department of Health and Human Services, Assistant Secretary for Legislation. 2002. "Statement by Joseph A. Levitt on Dietary Supplements and Their Use for Weight-Loss Purposes." Testimony before the Senate Committee on Governmental Affairs, Subcommittee on Oversight of Government Management, Restructuring, and the District of Columbia (31 July).

Hamilton, Kathryn K. 2001. "Antioxidant Supplements during Cancer Treatments: Where Do We Stand?" *Clinical Journal of Oncology Nursing* 5 (4): 181–182 (July/August).

Jacobs, Eric J. et al. 2002. "Vitamin C and Vitamin E Supplement Use and Bladder Cancer Mortality in a Large Cohort of US Men and Women." *American Journal of Epidemiology* 1;156 (11):1002–10 (December).

Labriola, Dan, and Robert Livingston. 1999. "Possible Interactions between Dietary Antioxidants and Chemotherapy." *Oncology* 13:1003–1011 (July).

Lamson Davis W., and Matthew S. Brignall. 1999. "Antioxidants in Cancer Therapy: Their Actions and Interactions with Oncologic Therapies." *Alternative Medicine Review* 4:304–329 (October).

Memorial Sloan-Kettering Cancer Center. 2003. AboutHerbs. Information Resource: AboutHerbs, Botanicals & Other Products. Available at: *http://www.mskcc.org/aboutherbs*.

Meyskens, Frank L. et al. 1994. "Randomized Trial of Vitamin A Versus Observation as Adjuvant Therapy in High-Risk Primary Malignant Melanoma: A Southwest Oncology Group Study." *Journal of Clinical Oncology* 12:2060–5 (October).

National Institutes of Health. 2002. Facts about Dietary Supplements (December). Available at: *http://www.cc.nih.gov/ccc/supplements*.

Oncolink. 2002. "Antioxidants during Chemotherapy." Ask the Experts. Abramson Cancer Center of the University of Pennsylvania (31 March).

Penland, James G. 2002. "Dietary Reference Intakes (DRIs): New Dietary Guidelines Really Are New!" Grand Forks Human Nutrition Research Center. United States Food and Drug Administration (12 April). Available at: *http://www.gfhnrc.ars.usda.gov/News/nws9912a.htm*.

Pure Prescriptions. 2003. "Prostate Product Review." Expert Opinions: Ask the Doctor. Available at: *http://www.pureprescriptions.com/expert_opinion/askthedoc/prostate_review.html*.

Stankiewicz, M. et al. 1989. "Complement Activation, Phagocytosis, Tumor Growth and Parasitic Infection after Magnesium Supplementation in Diet of Mice." *Magnesium* 8 (2):87–93.

United States Food and Drug Administration. 2001. "Illnesses and Injuries Associated With the Use of Selected Dietary Supplements." Center for Food Safety and Applied Nutrition (November). Available at: *http://vm.cfsan.fda.gov/~dms/ds-ill.html*.

United States Food and Drug Administration. 2001. "What Is a Dietary Supplement?" Food, Nutrition, and Cosmetics Questions & Answers (January). Available at: *http://www.cfsan.fda.gov/~dms/qa-sup5.html*.

Van Zandwijk, Nico et al. 2000. "EUROSCAN: A Randomized Trial of Vitamin A and N-Acetylcysteine in Patients with Head and Neck Cancer or Lung Cancer." *Journal of the National Cancer Institute* 92:977–86 (June).

Zeegers, Maurice P. A. et al. 2002. "Prediagnostic Toenail Selenium and Risk of Bladder Cancer." *Cancer Epidemiology Biomarkers & Prevention* 11 (11):1292–7 (November).

Chapter 6

Brown, Jean et al. 2001. "Nutrition During and After Cancer Treatment: A Guide for Informed Choices by Cancer Survivors." *CA: A Cancer Journal for Clinicians* 51:153–181 (May/June).

Cassileth, Barrie. *The Alternative Medicine Handbook.* New York: W.W. Norton & Company.

Memorial Sloan-Kettering Cancer Center. 2003. AboutHerbs. Information Resource: About Herbs, Botanicals & Other Products. Available at: *http://www.mskcc.org/aboutherbs*.

Chapter 7

Ghosh, Kris, Linda Carson, and Elyse Cohen. 2002. *Betty Crocker's Living with Cancer Cookbook.* New York: Hungry Minds.

National Cancer Institute. 1997. "Eating Hints for Cancer Patients: Before, During, and After Treatment." Available at: *http://www.cancer.gov/cancerinfo/eatinghints.*

National Cancer Institute. 2003. "Nutrition in Cancer Care." Physician Data Query. Available at: *http://www.nci. nih.gov/cancerinfo/pdq/supportivecare/nutrition/patient.*

Chapter 8

Brown, Jean et al. 2001. "Nutrition During and After Cancer Treatment: A Guide for Informed Choices by Cancer Survivors." *CA: A Cancer Journal for Clinicians* 51:153–181 (May/June).

Brown, Jean et al. 2003. "Nutrition and Physical Activity During and After Cancer Treatment: An American Cancer Society Guide for Informed Choices." *CA: A Cancer Journal for Clinicians* 53:268–291 (September/October).

National Cancer Institute. 1997. "Eating Hints for Cancer Patients: Before, During, and After Treatment." Available at: *http://www.cancer.gov/cancerinfo/eatinghints.*

Oncolink. 2001. "Liquid Nutrition Supplements." Ask the Experts. Abramson Cancer Center of the University of Pennsylvania (21 November).

Chapter 9

American Cancer Society. 2001. "Nutrition and Exercise Important After Treatment." ACS News Today (18 July). Available at: *http://www.cancer.org/docroot/NWS/content/ update/NWS_2_1xU_Nutrition_and_Exercise_Important_ After_Treatment_.asp.*

American Cancer Society. 2002. *Informed Decisions: The Complete Book of Cancer Diagnosis, Treatment, and Recovery.* Atlanta, Georgia: American Cancer Society.

Brown, Jean et al. 2001. "Nutrition During and After Cancer Treatment: A Guide for Informed Choices by Cancer Survivors." *CA: A Cancer Journal for Clinicians* 51:153–181 (May/June).

Brown, Jean et al. 2003. "Nutrition and Physical Activity During and After Cancer Treatment: An American Cancer Society Guide for Informed Choices." *CA: A Cancer Journal for Clinicians* 53:268–291 (September/October).

National Cancer Institute. 2003. "Nutrition in Cancer Care." Physician Data Query. Available at: *http://www.nci. nih.gov/cancerinfo/pdq/supportivecare/nutrition/patient.*

University of Michigan Comprehensive Cancer Center. 2003. "I Get Tired Easily." Managing Eating Problems. Available at: *http://www.cancer.med.umich.edu/learn/ nutrtired.htm.*

WebMD and the Cleveland Clinic. 2002. "Cancer-Related Fatigue." WebMD Condition Center. The Cleveland Clinic (April).

Chapter 10

Aker, Saundra N., and Polly Lenssen. 2000. *Guide to Good Nutrition during Cancer Therapy,* 4th ed. Seattle, Washington: Fred Hutchinson Cancer Research Center.

American Cancer Society. 2002. *American Cancer Society's Complementary and Alternative Cancer Methods Handbook.* Atlanta, Georgia: American Cancer Society.

American Cancer Society. 2003. "Impact of Altered Immune Function." Available at: *http://www.cancer.org/ docroot/PED/content/PED_3_2X_Impact_of_Altered_ Immune_Function.asp?sitearea=PED.*

American Dietetic Association. 2000. "The Clinical Guide to Oncology Nutrition: Patient Education Materials." Chicago, Illinois: American Dietetic Association.

Brown, Jean et al. 2001. "Nutrition During and After Cancer Treatment: A Guide for Informed Choices by Cancer Survivors." *CA: A Cancer Journal for Clinicians* 51:153–181 (May/June).

Chandra, R.K. 1997. "Nutrition and the Immune System: An Introduction." *American Journal of Clinical Nutrition* 66 (2):460S–463S (August).

Medline Plus Medical Information. 2002. "Exercise and Immunity." ADAM Medical Encyclopedia. Available at: *http://www.nlm.nih.gov/medlineplus/ency/article/007165.htm.*

National Institutes of Health. 2002. "NIH Funds Botanical Center in Iowa to Study Health Effects of Echinacea and St. John's Wort." News release (25 July).

Whitmire, Susan. 2000. Water, electrolytes, and acid-base balance. In *Krause's Food, Nutrition, and Diet Therapy,* 10th ed. L. Kathleen Mahan and Sylvia Escott-Stump. Philadelphia, Pennsylvania: W.B. Saunders and Company.

Chapter 11

Aker, Saundra N., and Polly Lenssen. 2000. *Guide to Good Nutrition during Cancer Therapy,* 4th ed. Seattle, Washington: Fred Hutchinson Cancer Research Center.

Bullers, Anne Christiansen. 2000. "Bottled Water: Better Than the Tap?" *FDA Consumer Magazine*. United States Food and Drug Administration. (July/August). Available at: *http://www.fda.gov/fdac/features/2002/402_h2o.html*.

Los Angeles Times. 2001. "All That Water Advice Just Doesn't Wash" (15 January).

National Cancer Institute. 1997. "Eating Hints for Cancer Patients: Before, During, and After Treatment." Available at: *http://www.cancer.gov/cancerinfo/eatinghints*.

National Cancer Institute. 2003. "Nutrition in Cancer Care." Physician Data Query. Available at: *http://www.cancer.gov/cancerinfo/pdq/supportivecare/nutrition/HealthProfessional#Section_157*.

Seattle Cancer Care Alliance. 2003. "Patient Diet and Nutrition Education Materials." Seattle, Washington: Clinical Nutrition and Patient Food Services Department.

Chapter 12

American Cancer Society. 2000. "Acupuncture Reduces Side Effects of Chemotherapy: Electroacupuncture Treatments Help Control Chemotherapy-related Vomiting." ACS News Today (27 December). Available at: *http://www.cancer.org/docroot/NWS/content/NWS_1_1x_Acupuncture_Reduces_Side_Effects_of_Chemotherapy.asp*.

American Dietetic Association. 2000. "The Clinical Guide to Oncology Nutrition: Patient Education Materials." Chicago, Illinois: American Dietetic Association.

Calhoun, Susan, and Jane Bradley. 1997. *Nutrition, Cancer and You*. Shawnee Mission, Kansas: Addax Publishing Group.

Goldwein, Joel W. 2001. "Chemotherapy for Patients: Introductory Information." Oncolink.com, Abramson Cancer Center of the University of Pennsylvania (November).

Margie, Joyce Daly, and Abby S. Bloch. 1984. *Nutrition and the Cancer Patient*. Radnor, Pennsylvania: Chilton Publishing.

Medline Plus Medical Information. 2002. "Lactose Intolerance." ADAM Medical Encyclopedia. Available at: *http://www.nlm.nih.gov/medlineplus/ency/article/000276.htm*.

National Cancer Institute. 1997. "Eating Hints for Cancer Patients: Before, During, and After Treatment." Available at: *http://www.cancer.gov/cancerinfo/eatinghints*.

National Cancer Institute. 2003. "Constipation." Physician Data Query. Available at: *http://www.nci.nih.gov/cancerinfo/pdq/supportivecare/constipation/patient*.

National Cancer Institute. 2003. "Nausea and Vomiting." Physician Data Query. Available at: *http://www.nci.nih.gov/cancerinfo/pdq/supportivecare/nausea/patient*.

National Cancer Institute. 2003. "Nutrition in Cancer Care." Physician Data Query. Available at: *http://www.nci.nih.gov/cancerinfo/pdq/supportivecare/nutrition/patient*.

National Cancer Institute. 2003. "Oral Complications." Physician Data Query. Available at: *http://www.nci.nih.gov/cancerinfo/pdq/supportivecare/oralcomplications/patient*.

National Comprehensive Cancer Network and the American Cancer Society. 2001. *Nausea and Vomiting: Treatment Guidelines for Patients with Cancer*. Version 1. Publication number 01-50M-No.9418-HCP (January).

United States Department of Agriculture. 2000. *The Report of the Dietary Guidelines Advisory Committee on the Dietary Guidelines for Americans*. Available at: *http://ars.usda.gov/dgac*.

University of Michigan Comprehensive Cancer Center. 2003. "Food Just Doesn't Taste the Same." Managing Eating Problems. Available at: *http://www.cancer.med.umich.edu/learn/nutrtastesame.htm*.

University of Michigan Comprehensive Cancer Center. 2003. "Loss of Appetite." Managing Eating Problems. Available at: *http://www.cancer.med.umich.edu/learn/nutrappetite.htm*.

Chapter 13

American Cancer Society. 1998. "The American Cancer Society's Skinny on Trimming the Fat." ACS News Today (24 February). Available at: *http://www.cancer.org/docroot/MED/content/MED_2_1X_The_American_Cancer_Society_s_Skinny_on_Trimming_the_Fat.asp*.

American Cancer Society. 1998. "Get Moving, at Any Age." ACS News Today (2 September). Available at: *http://www.cancer.org/docroot/NWS/content/NWS_2_1x_Get_moving__at_any_age.asp*.

American Cancer Society. 2001. "Nutrition and Exercise Important After Treatment." ACS News Today (18 July). Available at: *http://www.cancer.org/docroot/NWS/content/update/NWS_2_1xU_Nutrition_and_Exercise_Important_After_Treatment_.asp*.

American Cancer Society. 2003. "Controlling Portion Sizes." Available at: *http://www.cancer.org/docroot/PED/content/PED_3_2x_Portion_Control.asp*.

American Cancer Society. 2003. "Nutrition and Physical Activity Guidelines: Points to Remember." Available at: *http://www.cancer.org/docroot/SPC/content/SPC_1_Nutrition_and_Physical_Activity_Guidelines_Points_To_Remember.asp*.

American Cancer Society. 2003. "Restaurant Eating Tips." Available at: *http://www.cancer.org/docroot/PED/content/PED_3_2x_Restaurant_Eating_Tips_Mar_03.asp*.

American Cancer Society. 2004. *A Breast Cancer Journey: Your Personal Guidebook from the Experts at the American Cancer Society*, 2nd ed. Atlanta, Georgia: American Cancer Society.

American Institute of Cancer Research. 2002. "Survivors Guide: Understanding the Diet-Cancer Connection." Available at: *http://www.aicr.org/survivor*.

Brown, Jean et al. 2001. "Nutrition During and After Cancer Treatment: A Guide for Informed Choices by Cancer Survivors." *CA: A Cancer Journal for Clinicians* 51:153–181 (May/June).

Brown, Jean et al. 2003. "Nutrition and Physical Activity During and After Cancer Treatment: An American Cancer Society Guide for Informed Choices." *CA: A Cancer Journal for Clinicians* 53:268–291 (September/October).

Charity Wire. 2001. "At First-Ever Conference on Nutrition for Cancer Survivors, Researchers Vow to Find Needed Answers." Article 00244. American Institute for Cancer Research (8 May).

Holmes, Michelle D. et al. 1999. "Dietary Factors and the Survival of Women with Breast Carcinoma." *Cancer* 86:826–35 (November).

Maunsell, Elizabeth et al. 2002. "Dietary Change after Breast Cancer: Extent, Predictors, and Relation with Psychological Distress." *Journal of Clinical Oncology* 15;20(4):1017–25 (February).

National Cancer Institute. 1997. "Eating Hints for Cancer Patients: Before, During, and After Treatment." Available at: *http://www.cancer.gov/cancerinfo/eatinghints*.

Patterson, Ruth E. et al. 2003. "Changes in Diet, Physical Activity, and Supplement Use among Adults Diagnosed with Cancer." *Journal of the American Dietetic Association* 103 (3):323–8 (March).

UC Regents. 1998. "UC Davis Researchers Need Volunteers to Study Diet's Effects on Breast Cancer Recurrence." UC Davis News, Press Release (October 7). Available at: *http://news.ucdmc.ucdavis.edu/whelstudy.html*.

Young, Leslie R., and Marion Nestle. 2003. "Expanding Portion Sizes in the U.S. Marketplace: Implications for Nutrition Counseling." *Journal of the American Dietetic Association* 103 (2):231–4 (February).

Recipe Resource File

American Cancer Society. 2001. *American Cancer Society's Healthy Eating Cookbook: A Celebration of Food, Friends, and Healthy Living*. Second Edition. Atlanta, Georgia: American Cancer Society.

American Cancer Society. 2001. *Celebrate! Healthy Entertaining for Any Occasion*. Atlanta, Georgia: American Cancer Society.

National Cancer Institute. 1997. "Eating Hints for Cancer Patients: Before, During, and After Treatment." Available at: *http://www.cancer.gov/cancerinfo/eatinghints*.

Index

265